BIG
yoga

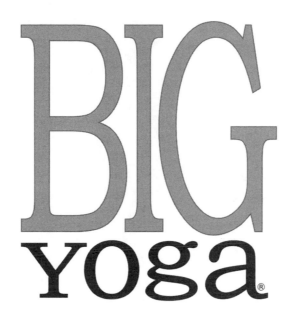

BIG Yoga®

A Simple Guide for Bigger Bodies

MEERA PATRICIA KERR

FOREWORD BY DEAN ORNISH, MD

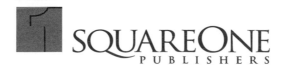

SQUAREONE
PUBLISHERS

As with any exercise program, consult with your doctor before beginning if you have questions or concerns. It is always better to err on the side of caution.

EDITOR: Anna Comstock
INDEXER: Caryn Woerner
COVER DESIGNER: Jeannie Tudor
TYPESETTER: Gary A. Rosenberg
COVER AND INTERIOR PHOTO CREDIT: Tim LaDuke of LaDuke Studios
(www.ladukestudios.com)

Square One Publishers
115 Herricks Road
Garden City Park, NY 11040
(516) 535-2010 • (877) 900-BOOK
www.squareonepublishers.com

Poem on dedication page from "Like a Hobo-Gobu" by Patricia Kerr. Copyright © 1975 ColleyWabbles Music. Reprinted by permission.

Library of Congress Cataloging-in-Publication Data
Kerr, Meera Patricia.
 Big yoga : a simple guide for bigger bodies / Meera Patricia Kerr.
   p. cm.
 ISBN 978-0-7570-0215-1
 1. Yoga. 2. Overweight persons—Health and hygiene. I. Title.
 RA781.7.K47 2009
 613.7'046—dc22

2009043139

Printed in Canada

10   9   8   7   6   5   4   3   2

Contents

To my beautiful Guru,
His Holiness Sri Swami Satchidananda

"I offer it all unto to you Lord,
Knowing everything I have is Thine
Won't you be my constant companion?
Show me the light, Let me shine."

Acknowledgments

Over the thirty or so years that I've been studying and practicing Yoga, I have met many wonderful Yoga teachers to whom I am deeply grateful—from the great Sri Swami Satchidananda and his ancient lineage, to his assistant Dr. Prem Anjali, to the entire Integral Yoga organization. Thanks also to Mukunda Styles, Hope Mell, and other dear sangha members and teachers too numerous to mention.

Additionally, I would like to extend a thank you to my family—especially Sam and Dave Alexander, who came to live with me at Yogaville so I could be immersed in the Yogic life. Thanks also to their father, Lester Sukarta Alexander, who helped me shape the first draft of this book and gave me unfailing encouragement.

I am indebted to Rick Rosenthal who produced my first *Big Yoga* DVD, and to Christine McMahan who has provided all the artwork for Big Yoga Media, including the wonderful logo.

A special thanks also goes to Ganesh MacIsaac at Integral Yoga Distribution, who led me to Square One Publishers, and to publisher Rudy Shur, who "got it" about *Big Yoga*. Rudy spent many hours helping me shape the manuscript, ably assisted by Anna Comstock and Jeannie Tudor. I also want to thank Tim LaDuke for making my photo shoot for the book effortless and fun.

Finally, I am profoundly grateful for the students who have come to *Big Yoga* for healing and renewal. Thank you all for allowing me to be of service.

Foreword

I first met Meera in 1978 at the Satchidananda Ashram in Connecticut, where I had just given a talk on the encouraging results of a medical research study I had conducted. My colleagues and I had been able to demonstrate that patients with severe heart disease could begin to reverse their condition through the use of yoga, meditation, improved nutrition, moderate exercise, and other comprehensive lifestyle changes.

At the end of my talk, Meera and her husband, Les Alexander, came up to me. Les said, "You should write a book!" He offered to introduce me to some of his friends in the publishing business, and they invited me to come to Manhattan to stay with them at their mid-town apartment. The result of our meeting was the publication of my first book, *Stress, Diet, and Your Heart*.

Over these many years, the work I have been directing at the non-profit Preventive Medicine and Research Institute has proven the efficacy of the techniques of yoga for managing stress and promoting heath and healing. While my original research was aimed at patients suffering from severe heart disease, the lifestyle changes that were offered in the medical trials are equally applicable to other health challenges.

In a series of randomized controlled trials and demonstration projects, we found that comprehensive lifestyle changes, including yoga, may stop or even reverse the progression of coronary heart disease, early-stage prostate cancer, type 2 diabetes, high blood pressure, high cholesterol levels, and obesity.

Our latest studies showed that these lifestyle changes may even alter genes—"turning on" genes that prevent chronic diseases and "turning off" oncogenes that promote breast cancer and prostate cancer. They may also turn off genes that cause inflammation and oxidative stress, which may be root causes of heart disease and other illnesses.

Meera's *Big Yoga* is a comprehensive program that provides both yoga postures adapted to the larger body, as well as other important elements of yoga philosophy, including meditation, devotion, and introspection. Her approach is gentle and compassionate, encouraging people who may have felt they really didn't belong in a yoga class to give yoga a try.

Big Yoga is a wonderful introduction to the ancient art and science of yoga for those challenged by extra weight, stiffness, injury, or disabilities. It is a welcome addition to the bounty of yoga books available today.

Dean Ornish M.D.
Founder and President, Preventive Medicine Research Institute
Clinical Professor of Medicine, University of California, San Francisco
www.pmri.org

Introduction

When I started studying Yoga, I was always the most "well-rounded" person in the room. My Yoga teachers were, without exception, slender, graceful, soft-spoken, and flexible. I, on the other hand, was beefy, athletic, and loud. Even though I was as flexible as everyone else, it was clear I was of a different body type. Surprisingly, though, it didn't bother me! The benefits of Yoga class far exceeded any embarrassment I may have had.

I was used to being different. I grew up getting criticized for being fat by my mother, who never had a weight problem, and ridiculed by my brother, who liked to call me "Fattie Pattie"—the name of a pop song from the 1950's. My father was more understanding because my body fit the template of all his relatives, who were, in the words of the day, "heavy-set." And I, for some mysterious reason, had a certain obliviousness to the negativity around my size, even as a child. It's not that it didn't hurt to be singled out, even taunted by people of normal weight, but I always had a feeling it was their problem, not mine.

What a blessing. And it really was a blessing, a natural grace, rather than something I had to figure out or earn for myself. I just came that way. Similarly, I never had any fear of singing or performing in public, and was the unrivaled choice for star of the kindergarten musical. I still love getting up in front of people and sharing my passions. If I didn't, I could never have allowed myself to be photographed for this book in revealing positions and outfits!

I stopped going to the gym years ago because I felt so out of place, but I still wanted to stay fit. If you, like me, are a curvy-girl or a hefty-man, you may also be looking for an exercise program that allows you to accept your body as it is right now. It is possible to be fit and fat! In fact, research shows that a healthy person of size has a better chance at longevity than a thinner person who is out of shape.

Big Yoga is a fitness program that offers adaptations to traditional Yoga poses, making them accessible to all people including those challenged by weight, stiffness, age, or disabilities. The simple act of breathing and stretching with mindful awareness—which you'll learn about later—is the key. In fact, you can even get benefits from a Yoga video simply by watching it with full attention, so imagine how great you'll feel if you actually do it!

There is more to Yoga than just the physical postures, but the poses, traditionally called *asanas,* provide a good point of entry into the path of health and self-discovery. *Big Yoga* offers a smorgasbord of different techniques and approaches that appeal to different styles of learning and transformation. As you begin your own Yoga practice, you may find yourself attracted to the exercises, but gradually, you may be drawn toward Yoga's other, more meditative aspects.

I've been teaching Yoga for over thirty years and have watched my body change with the cycles of life: young and voluptuous, pregnant and plump, postpartum and nursing, struggling to get back in shape, menopausal and cranky. Now, I seem to have settled into older and wiser. I have realized the need to modify my personal practice to bring myself more ease and comfort, to accommodate my own soft curves, and to bring the maximum benefit to my body. Though I am constantly changing, my Yoga practice grounds me in self-care, and my meditations help me to accept the eccentricities of nature.

If you have a body that looks more like mine than, say, Charlize Theron's, Kelly Rippa's, or Will Smith's, then *Big Yoga* is for you. Its gentle stretches will increase your flexibility and muscle tone. And practicing it regularly will help turn your mind inward to the peace within. This meditative awareness is a powerful tool in reducing stress.

WHAT YOU WILL FIND IN THIS BOOK

Over the thirty-five or so years that I've been studying Yoga, I've accumulated a vast amount of practical knowledge, hard-won experience, and numerous books, tapes, and CDs. I was privileged to sit at the feet of my own teacher, His Holiness Sri Swami Satchidananda—who we called Swamiji, and later, Gurudev—and humbly listen to his inspiring lectures on the day-to-day application of Yoga philosophy. Swamiji could not only speak on Yoga, he was a living embodiment of the goal of Yoga: to realize the Truth within. Yoga is a deep subject, and I find myself going back to the well time and time again. Hopefully, a little of Swamiji's spirit has been imparted to me and I, in turn, can share it with you. This book is a refinement of all I have learned, and my hope is that it makes Yoga accessible to everyone.

Part One will ease you into Yoga by giving you some historical background information, as well as some preparatory tips. You will learn about props and equipment that you can buy to assist you with your practice, as well as alternatives that you might already have lying around the house! Additionally, you will learn that everyone encounters stumbling blocks and has days when their motivation is lacking—you are not alone! We all struggle to find the time to take good care of ourselves. However, this book will teach you how to handle and overcome those situations so you can continue on your path toward health.

Part Two is where the Yoga exercises are explained and demonstrated. It starts out with the physical postures (what most people think of when they think of Yoga), and then moves into the deeper Yogic practices of breathing, meditation, service, and devotion. Throughout, you will find a blend of information for beginners, interspersed with more advanced ideas to hold your interest as you become more experienced. Thus, regardless of your ability level, you will find the information you need to be successful.

HOW TO USE THIS BOOK

You can use this book in many ways, so choose the one that works best for you. If you're a kinesthetic learner, that is, someone who learns in a physical way, you might want to skip all the preliminary information in Part One and jump right into the physical poses, which are pictured and explained in Part Two. However, if you learn more readily through words and language, you may be more comfortable reading the entire book cover-to-cover first, and then going back to the section on asanas. If you're a visual learner, you may discover that watching Yoga movements on a DVD is easiest for you. If that is the case, I suggest you check out the *Big Yoga Hatha One* DVD, which offers a gentle adapted Yoga practice that you can do in the privacy of your own home (see page 210 for details), and simply use this book as a supplement.

Regardless of how you use it, though, there is a depth to Yoga that will keep you coming back to this book as your primary resource. It's all right here! Whether you're a beginner to Yoga or have tried it in the past (and maybe gotten discouraged), *Big Yoga* has something for everyone. Incorporating it into your daily routine can truly change your life on many different levels. So, let's get started!

Part One

Yoga Basics

The material in this first part discusses everything from the history of Yoga, to Yoga's health benefits, to the equipment you will need to get started in your own practice. Yoga comes from a long lineage that goes back thousands of years. In the beginning, all Yogic wisdom was handed down from teacher to student in an oral tradition. In fact, the teachings had actually been around for hundreds of years before they were compiled and put on paper—well, originally, on palm leaves. In the first chapter, we'll learn about the history of Yoga, including how it evolved as it moved out of India and into all the corners of the Earth.

In chapter two, we delve deep into the benefits of Yoga. It's amazing to me that the ancient Yogis had strategies for keeping the entire bodily system in balance without the aide of today's modern medical technology. This, alone, is a great reason to begin practicing Yoga! Yogic solutions to whatever issues you may be dealing with are discussed and explained. This chapter is all about you and your body, and I hope you will find it inspiring!

In the third chapter, we spell out all the necessary items you will need in order to enjoy your Yoga practice. You can keep it bare bones with just a towel and a pillow, or you can go all out and buy mats, blocks, and other props. Later in the chapter, we offer tips on getting the most out of your practice, including a short section on Yogic diet. And we also stress the need to have compassionate self-acceptance as you begin. When we use this powerful, positive attitude during our practice, it will gradually become a way of life.

Finally, in chapter four we offer some solutions to common stumbling blocks. If you find it hard to get yourself on a regular Yoga schedule, know that you're not alone—that's why ashrams were invented! When apathy or busy schedules strike, remember that you don't have to do every pose, every day, and sit for meditation twice a day! You will notice the benefits by simply adding a little Yoga into your daily life, whatever you have time for. It's great to have lofty goals, but don't get discouraged if you initially fall short of meeting them. Keep plugging along and you will eventually get to where you want to go. It's a wonderful journey, and it's time to begin!

Chapter 1

The Evolution of Yoga

My first exposure to Yoga happened back in the 1960's. My college roommate brought a Yoga book, which was yellow with age and had rarely been checked out of the library, back to our dorm room. Both of us quickly became fascinated by the pictures in it, which were of an exotic-looking young man wearing what looked like a diaper! (I've since learned that this is a common Indian garb, called a *dhoti*.) We passed the book around to several other giggling girls, who, like us, poured over the photographs of the young man performing extraordinary feats of flexibility and strength. I only had a brief look at the book before it went back to the lonely stacks at the library, but somehow, subconsciously, I was hooked on Yoga.

The word *Yoga* comes from the Sanskrit root word *yug*, meaning to yoke or unite. Through the practice of exercise and breathing, Yoga unites our bodies, minds, and spirits, and brings us into a state of balance; it makes us feel still, renewed, and refreshed. Interestingly, the root word of *religion* has a similar meaning: to bind or connect. Although Yoga is not a religion, after practicing its exercises and breathing techniques, we connect to our higher selves. And when we come together to do Yoga, there is an added benefit of connecting with each other and creating community.

Perhaps your first connection to Yoga, similar to my own, is from the numerous pictures and articles about it—usually portraying lean, lithe, young lovelies performing extreme postures in body-hugging outfits—that are sprinkled throughout the media. These images make Yoga look cool, and the pictures in my oodles of books on Yoga mostly depict this same body type. But that doesn't tell the whole story. Today, there is a need for more variety—for other options that can work for our bodies as they are now. That is why I have put together *Big Yoga*. Before we begin, though, it's important to take a minute to learn about where Yoga came from, as well as what other movements throughout history it has impacted.

YOGA'S ORIGINATION

We don't know the exact origin of Yoga, but we do know that it emerged at least 5,000 years ago in the Indus Valley—now called India. As civilization was getting its act together during the Bronze Age—beginning around 3300 BCE—several important Hindu texts emerged, including the Bhagavad Gita. These ancient Yoga works were written in the Sanskrit language, which is the classical language of India. In one such scripture, it states simply, "Yoga is ecstasy."

Later, around 200 BCE, another important text called the *Yoga Sutras* emerged. It was written on palm leaves and contained 195 sutras—*sutra* meaning thread, as in just a thread of an idea. These pithy sutras were part of an oral tradition going back hundreds, even thousands of years. The sage Patanjali—commonly referred to as the father of modern Yoga—purportedly compiled the text, which forms the basis of what is today known as Raja Yoga, or, the royal path of Yoga. The text lays out the basics of Yoga theory, asserting it to be a state of blissful consciousness beyond the mind, and offers a variety of practices for calming the mind in order to achieve that state.

By the time Patanjali had compiled the *Yoga Sutras*, the teachings of Yoga had already begun to spread from India to other parts of the Eastern world. As Yogis moved into Pakistan, their Yoga continued to evolve and it may have become the basis of Sikhism. Yoga influenced other religions as it spread throughout Asia, as well, including Buddhism, Zen, Jainism, and Confucianism.

Politics, world affairs, and even money have also had a hand in the evolution of Yoga. Indian culture began to have an impact on the West because of trade. Do you remember studying about the East India Company in grade school? Me neither, so here's a little refresher. In 1600, a conglomeration of British merchants who were involved in trading with the Far East, brought treasures such as cotton, silk, indigo dye, and of course, tea, back to England. What started out as a commercial venture ended up in a power struggle, with the British assuming control of the Indian government and military. If you've seen the movie *Gandhi* you already know how this story ends. For those of you who haven't, India struggled for its independence from Britain, finally achieving it in 1950.

Cotton and silks weren't the only items of value to reach Britain from India— Yoga did, too! In the 1800's, the British head of state, Queen Victoria, boldly took the title of Empress of India. Her interest in Indian things led to a fascination with Yoga, and Yogis from India were brought to court to perform for her amusement. Imagine the Queen, all gussied up, watching a scantily clad Yogi walk over coals, stand on his head, or rest on a bed of nails. Today, these images seem like harmless cartoons, but in the prim and proper Victorian era, seeing a half-dressed man was shocking!

And so, although it was probably for all the wrong reasons, Yoga captured the imaginations of the rich and powerful. It was something new, interesting, and a little freaky, too. However, beyond the fascination with the Yogis' bizarre antics, there was a genuine interest in the way they had supreme control of their bodies. From then on, Yoga's influence continued to spread.

EAST/WEST FUSION

Yoga had arrived in Europe and Asia, and it eventually found its way to the United States near the end of the nineteenth century. In 1893, the eloquent Swami Vivekananda came to Chicago from India to speak at the Parliament of Religions—a conference held as part of the Columbian Exposition (an early World's Fair). This interfaith event marked the earliest formal gathering of representatives of Eastern and Western spiritual traditions from around the world. It was also the first opportunity Americans had to meet an authentic Yoga master and discuss the lofty ideals of various religious traditions.

The Exposition had a profound impact on the 27 million people who attended. It displayed an incredible array of architectural styles, all done in faux white marble, as well as a dazzling, extravagant display of electric lights, which were still a novelty to many at the time. It also gave attendees the opportunity to overlook the whole fair from the top of the world's first Ferris wheel, with views of Lake Michigan and acres of lush landscaping by the eminent Frederick Law Olmsted, creator of New York's Central Park. Chicago, and Midwesterners in general who were considered "hayseeds" by many from the bigger, more sophisticated cities like Paris and New York, would never be the same!

I know this sounds like it happened more than a hundred years ago (Oh, I guess it did . . .), but believe it or not, my great-grandmother Henrietta was living in Chicago at the time and she attended the conference! In fact, a few summers ago as I was cleaning our summer cottage, which had originally belonged to her, I discovered a book on Yoga in her library and a program from the conference underneath a stack of linens and organ music at the bottom of her trunk. Imagine that! I had a Yogi-granny!

In 1920, another great Indian Yogi came to America: Paramahansa Yogananda. Growing up in India under British Rule gave him a command of the English language, as well as an affinity for the Western way of thinking. He also had a love of chanting and traveled around the country sharing his self-penned *bhajans,* or devotional songs—many of them written in English with an Indian flavor. His *Autobiography of a Yogi,* published in 1946, is still one of the bestselling books on Yoga.

THE BACK TO NATURE MOVEMENT

Throughout the early twentieth century, interest in Yoga—sparked by the World Parliament of Religions—began to permeate into the minds of creative people who had their own ideas about health and fitness. Take, for instance, Dr. John H. Kellogg. It's hard for some people to imagine a morning without corn flakes, but they were unknown until they were marketed by Dr. Kellogg in 1894.

In addition to breakfast cereals, Kellogg's interest in health and natural cures inspired him to open the Battle Creek Sanitarium in Michigan in the early 1900's. His sanitarium was known for its emphasis on many of the same things that were espoused in Yoga: sunbathing, vegetarian diet, exercise, and enemas! He even invented his own device for colon cleansing. Kellogg, like the Yogis, believed the body was a living temple. He also believed the colon was the seat of most disease in the body, and therefore, it should be kept clean from above and below. As I studied up on Kellogg, I couldn't help wondering if he had associated with the Yogis at the Exposition in Chicago, because there is a striking similarity to his theories on colon health and the ancient Yoga texts on *basti*—a type of primitive enema. You can learn more about Kellog's bizarre ways in the quirky movie, *The Road to Wellville*, starring John Cusak, Anthony Hopkins, Bridget Fonda, and Matthew Broderick.

One of Kellogg's protégés was Jethro Kloss, author of *Back to Eden*, a classic in the fields of herbal medicines, natural foods, and home remedies. It has been a consistent bestseller since its publication in 1939. As the title indicates, Kloss was encouraging a return to natural cures in response to what he saw as the unpleasant, and sometimes disastrous, effects of the drugs that were being prescribed by medical doctors of the day. The booming natural foods industry of today owes a tip of the hat to Jethro Kloss!

Dr. Bernard Jensen, a chiropractor from California, took up where Kellogg left off. In the early 1930's, he started his own sanitariums, which focused on fasting, detoxing, and juice therapy. He also wrote several books on these subjects, including a natural guide to weight control. As a beginning student of Yoga, my teachers exposed me to the books written by Kloss and Dr. Jensen. And many of us practicing Yoga in the 1970's were experimenting with fasting—using the bentonite, apple juice, and psylliym seed cocktail that helped to purge the body of toxins supposedly left over from a lifetime of eating meat, white flour, and white sugar. I can speak from experience that fasting can rejuvenate the body, but it requires a lot of focus and preparation. You can't just stop eating, and it isn't recommended for anyone who tends toward bulimia or anorexia.

Another early health entrepreneur, Paul Bragg, wrote a health column for the Los Angeles Times in the 1920's. The column expounded on his beliefs that deep breathing, fasting, juicing, and eating organic foods were the way to a long and healthy life. It's not clear whether he got his ideas about deep breathing and fasting from Yoga, but many of them seem as if they sprung from the deep well of Yogic wisdom. Bragg toured the country promoting his books and giving lectures and private consultations. One of his followers is the amazing Jack LaLanne, born in 1914, who claims he can't afford to die because it would ruin his reputation! Although we may think of LaLanne essentially as a body builder, he is also into juicing, and you may have seen his infomercials on his own brand of power juicer.

So, we have two parallel universes here. Did the interest in Yoga flourish because of the simultaneous interest in natural health remedies? Or, were the ideas expounded by Dr. Jensen, Dr. Kellogg, and others a natural evolution of thought, stemming from an interest in Yoga? The answer probably lies somewhere between the two trains of thought. Regardless, Yoga and health were thriving. And whatever you may say about these health-nuts, you have to admit, they were onto something. LaLanne is pushing 100, Dr. Kellogg lived to 91, Dr. Jensen to 93, and Kloss to 84. Paul Bragg, at 76, was the youngest to pass away, but he did so from complications after a surfing accident, not because his health failed him.

WOODSTOCK RESURGENCE

After flourishing during the back-to-nature movement in the early part of the twentieth century, interest in Yoga and health waned somewhat—probably because America was busy fighting World Wars and recovering economically from the stock market crash of 1929. However, a resurgence in the mind-body field occurred in the 1960's and early 70's, when a host of Indian Yoga masters came to America to lecture and demonstrate the Yogic lifestyle.

Hippies and freaks, disgusted with the Vietnam War machine and the complicity of their parents' generation, were looking for a different way of thinking and living. And then, in 1969, Woodstock happened and their wish was granted. It was one of the earliest large-scale events celebrating the counter-culture. My teacher, Sri Swami Satchidananda, is known as the "Woodstock Swami," because he was invited to open the event with simple peace chants, setting the tone for the entire wild weekend.

Swami Satchidananada sat on the stage in traditional Indian garb, beard and long hair flowing, looking very much like a hippie himself. He had come to the states in 1966 at the request of the artist, Peter Max. He was originally only going to visit for a few days and teach Yoga to Peter and some of his friends, but they begged him to stay. So, what started as a short visit became a life's work, bringing his Integral Yoga to the West.

Swami Satchidananda's brother monk, Swami Vishnu-Devananda, came to Canada in 1966—around the same time that Swami Satchidananda came to New

York. They were both students of Swami Sivananda, who, before his death in 1963, had urged them to bring Yoga to the West. It is purported that Swami Sivananda said to Swami Vishnu-Devananada, "People are waiting!" It seemed as if Swami Sivananda knew Westerners were waiting to learn the ancient wisdom of Yoga!

Swami Vishnu-Devananda began teaching the Sivananda style Yoga, first in Canada, and later in the United States. Other Yoga teachers who came to the West in the 1960's were Swami Rama of the Himalayan Institute, Yogi Bhajan of the

---

His Holiness Sri Swami Satchidananda

The Reverend Sri Swami Satchidananda—known as Swamiji, and later, Gurudev—was born on December 22, 1914 in a small village in South India. Even as a child he had a devotional nature, which was encouraged by his highly spiritual family. As a young adult, he worked in the fields of agriculture, mechanics, electronics, and cinematography. Later, he turned his attention to serious spiritual practice and studied with many great spiritual masters, including Sri Ramana Maharshi and Sri Aurobindo. When he met His Holiness Sri Swami Sivananda of the Divine Life Society in Rishikesh, he knew he had found his mentor and guru. He received initiation into the Paramahamsa Order of Sannyas in 1949, and spent the rest of his life sharing his

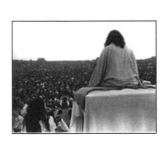
Swami Satchidananda
at Woodstock

vast knowledge of Yoga and serving others, first in India, later in the U.S., and ultimately all over the world.

Before his death in 2002, Swami Satchidananda accomplished many things. He founded the Integral Yoga Institutes in 1966 to spread the ancient teachings of Yoga. Additionally, in 1983 he established the Light of Truth Universal Shrine (LOTUS), dedicated to the Light of all faiths and to world peace at the Sachidananda Ashram in Yogaville, Virginia. Yogaville is the culmination of his vision for a "heaven on earth." It's a place where people of all faiths and backgrounds can come to study and practice the principles of Integral Yoga.

Swami Satchidananda took Mahasamadhi —a God-realized soul's conscious exit from the body—on August 19, 2002 in South India. His life-long message emphasized harmony among people of all races and faiths, and his motto was: "Truth is One, Paths are Many." During his life, he was awarded the Martin Buber Award for Outstanding Service to Humanity, the B'nai Brith Anti-Defamation League's Humanitarian Award, and the Albert Schweitzer Humanitarian award. His body is enshrined in Yogaville at the Chidambaram Shrine, which is open to the public for prayer and meditation.

His Holiness Sri Swami Sivananda

Born Kuppuswami on September 8, 1887 in South India, Sivananda was a vigorous and intelligent child. He attended medical school, and after graduation he practiced medicine for ten years, often deferring fees for those who couldn't afford his care. In his late thirties, he began to feel a strong pull for the renounced life, so he moved to Rishikesh, where he met his guru, Swami Vishwananda Saraswati. He was initiated into the Sannyas order and given the name Sivananda. He practiced intense spiritual practices while continuing to help the sick.

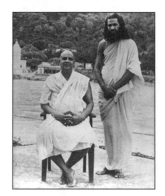

H.H. Sri Swami Sivananda (seated)

Swami Sivananda is the author of over 300 books on spiritual life, and he founded the Divine Life Society on the banks of the Ganges River. He also created the Sivananda Ayurvedic Pharmacy and organized the All-World Religions Federations. Swami Sivananda was devoted to the idea of the essential oneness of all religions, and his philosophy can be summed up in his famous sutra: Serve, Love, Give, Purify, Meditate, Realize!

Kundalini Yoga tradition, Amrit Desai from Kripalu, and Swami Muktananda of the Siddha Yoga tradition.

B.K.S. Iyengar, possibly the best known of all the Hatha Yoga teachers, has rarely been to the United States, but is well known as a teacher of teachers. Many of his students promote the Iyengar tradition through their books, tapes, and DVDs, including Rodney Yee, Suzanne Deason, and Patricia Walden. This was the first wave of the Yoga renaissance that began in America in the 1960's, and then, oddly enough, worked its way back to India, where many Western Yoga teachers have been called to teach.

Although Iyengar's teacher, T. Krishnamacharya, never came to the United States himself, he deserves a mention here. Considered by many to be the "Grandfather of Modern Yoga," Krishnamacharya was also teacher to other famous contemporary Yoga students and teachers, such as Indra Devi, Pattabhi Jois, and Krishnamacharya's son, T.K.V. Desikachar.

Today's modern Yoga is an offshoot of classical Indian Yoga tradition. We literally have hundreds of types of Yoga being practiced in community centers, YMCA's, gyms, and Yoga studios all over America. Yoga is now a part of the American culture, we have made it our own, and it is the perfect antidote to the stressful, twenty-first century lifestyle.

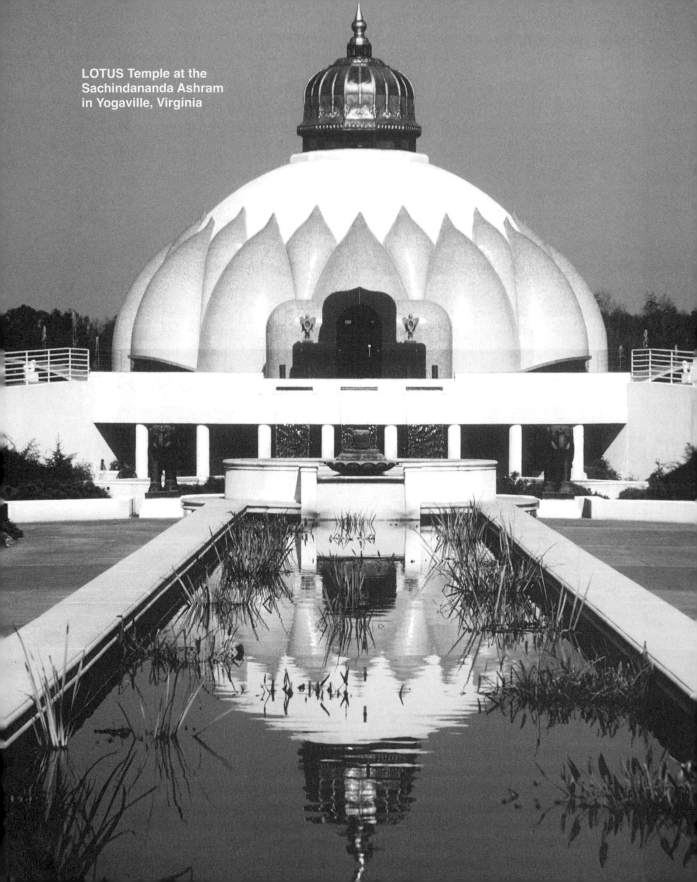

LOTUS Temple at the Sachindananda Ashram in Yogaville, Virginia

HATHA YOGA

Yoga has become mainstream, and Hatha Yoga, in particular, is its calling card. Hatha is one of several systems of Yoga, and it includes physical postures (*asanas*), breathing exercises (*pranayama*), and cleansing practices (*kriyas*). The word *Hatha* is combination of two ancient Sanskrit words—*ha*, meaning sun (sometimes referred to as the warming or masculine side), and *tha*, meaning moon (sometimes referred to as the cooling, more receptive, feminine side). Together, *Hatha* represents the right and left sides of the body, respectively, as well as energy patterns throughout the body, called *nadis*. Hatha Yoga attempts to create a balance between mind, body, and these subtle energies. Regular Hatha practice also helps focus the mind, raises self-confidence, and improves mood. Over time, the physical postures begin to regulate the entire body, giving it strength, flexibility, and vitality.

When most people think of Yoga, they typically conjure an image of someone in a leotard performing a Hatha pose. In fact, the physical postures are probably what you're hoping to learn from this book. (And don't worry, they are coming in Part Two!) Although the physical postures and breathing practices are the aspects of Yoga most commonly practiced in the United States, they are only two of the eight branches of the virtual Yoga tree that comprises Patanjali's Raja Yoga system. See page 179 for more information about the tree of Yoga.

These two important branches focus on making the body fit for meditation and even higher states of consciousness, called *samadhi*—the ultimate goal of Yoga. When the body is out of shape and full of aches and pains, it's almost impossible to sit for long periods without squirming, which doesn't lead to a very tranquil meditation. And it's difficult to evolve into higher states of awareness when we're hung-up on the body. Part Two of this book, beginning on page 43, details the practices of Hatha's physical postures, breathing exercises, and meditation techniques. In addition, Part Two also touches on Bhakti Yoga, the devotional aspect; Karma Yoga, the path of selfless service; and Jnana Yoga, the path of wisdom and self-analysis.

THE DEVELOPMENT OF *BIG YOGA*

It seems that I was destined to be a Big Yogi. I grew up plump but flexible, and I enjoyed moving, especially swimming, hiking, and dancing. I was also attracted to the spiritual, having grown up as a chorister in the Episcopal Church. I was often transported by the celestial music we performed. And as a child of the 1960's, I naturally gravitated to all things hippie, including Yoga.

I began studying Yoga in earnest when I was living in Connecticut. I was in the process of putting together an all-female band there, when Swami

Satchidananda came to our small Yoga center in Danbury. After meeting him, we all became *Gurubhais,* or devotees. From the beginning, I had a strong feeling that everything I needed to know about Yoga I could learn from this man, so I decided to go to a silent, ten-day Yoga retreat, where I could receive *mantra* initiation from Swamiji himself. A few years later, I took teacher training and began teaching at the Integral Yoga Institute in New York, because I wanted to share Yoga with others.

Fast-forward to the early 1990's. I was living at the Sachidananda Ashram in Central Virginia in a magical place called Yogaville. Yogaville is the home of Swami Sachidananda's Integral Yoga organization. I was drawn to studying Integral Yoga because it doesn't just focus on Yoga's physical side. It is more about bringing Yoga into all aspects of our lives—the way we act, speak, and think. Additionally, the concepts of non-violence, purity, and contentment create an element of grace in the teachers and students of Integral Yoga.

That being said, I, personally, never really bought into the name. As a songwriter, I didn't like the sound of the word "integral." It was hard to pronounce and some people didn't know what it meant. Then, one day while walking to noon meditation at the LOTUS Temple—I was pondering the questions: "Is there another way to express the concept of Integral Yoga? What's another way to say the same thing?"

As I settled into my silent meditation, I heard a voice say, "Big Yoga." I was struck with the happy realization that this was the answer to my questions. *Big,* as in expansive and inclusive of all the various Yoga practices, but also *big* in terms of the body: a comprehensive Yoga for bigger people. I knew of Swami Satchidananda's love of word-play and felt that this message, with its delightful double-entendre, had come directly from him. If you get any benefit from *Big Yoga,* I defer much of the credit to the teachings of Integral Yoga and the incomparable Sri Swami Satchidananda.

Chapter 2

What Yoga Can Do for You

Today, Yoga is a booming American business. There are over 15.8 million people practicing Yoga in this country alone. And not only can you can find Yoga classes in just about every city and town, you can also find Yoga DVDs, retreats, mats, props, music, clothing, eye pillows, meditation pillows, and fitness magazines with pictures of buff athletes doing extreme poses. However, even amongst all of this variety and exposure, you may still be wondering, *"Is there anything out there for me? Can I do Yoga?"* The answer is a resounding, *"Yes!"*

Today, what we think of as Yoga are primarily the physical postures, or *asanas*. Maharishi Patanjali, compiler of the *Yoga Sutras*, defined asana as any steady, comfortable posture. However, some of the traditional asanas are not comfortable for everyone! I've been teaching and studying Yoga for over thirty years, and as I got a little older, I realized that different bodies are comfortable doing different things. I found a need to modify my personal practice to accommodate my own soft curves and to bring more ease, comfort, and benefit to my body—thus fulfilling the true definition of asana. Therefore, I developed *Big Yoga*, which takes traditional physical postures and adapts them with larger bodies in mind.

Though I may not fit the physical description of the classic Yoga teacher, I have maintained my good health even into my sixties. I am passionate about Yoga's healing effects and want to share my practice with others—those who want to try Yoga but might not feel comfortable in public classes because of their size or lack of flexibility. As long as you have breath in your body, you can benefit from *Big Yoga*.

So, forget the pictures you have seen of the super flexible Yoga models twisted into various positions. If a position isn't comfortable for you, it isn't Yoga. And although Yoga is often practiced on the floor using a towel or a mat, you will soon learn that it can also be effectively practiced while sitting on a chair, standing, or even lying in a bed—whatever works best for you.

WHY YOGA IS IMPORTANT TO DAILY LIFE

What is creating stress in your life? It could be that you're challenged by working a full-time job and raising children at the same time. Maybe you're the caretaker of an elderly family member. Or, you might be dealing with your own health problems or financial worries. Any way you look at it, twenty-first century life has become increasingly stressful. Stress has a hand in many of today's biggest health problems, including diseases common to people who are overweight. When we are under stress, our cortisol—the stress hormone—levels become elevated, leaving us at risk for higher blood-sugar levels, higher blood pressure, and higher triglycerides. Elevated cortisol also lowers bone density and is linked to insulin resistance—a precursor to diabetes.

Thankfully, we have a way out of this stress cycle. We may not have control over the challenging events in our lives, but with practice, we can make choices about how we react to stress. Yoga trains the body to relax, and the effects can be felt after just one session. Many of my new students are amazed by how relaxed they feel at the end of their first class, as if they had forgotten what it even feels like to really let go. With regular practice, the body can return to this feeling of relaxation more readily. As we begin to gain more control over the body, the mind will follow. And with the mind under our control, we can slow down our reaction time to stressful events. Over time, this control permeates our daily lives, and our minds become our allies instead of our enemies.

You may have heard the phrase, "The body is a temple." It means that since we're going to spend our lives existing in our bodies, we should treat them with care and respect. Yoga can help us do that by moving us out of the rat race and into the sacred. During the practice of Yoga, vital energies are recycled and enhanced, toxins are released and cleared out of the body, and negative thoughts are purged from the mind. It brings us into a greater alignment with our authentic selves. In short, Yoga can help us become, in the words of author Eckart Tolle, "A blessing on the earth, and not a burden."

THE POWERFUL BENEFITS OF YOGA

Traditional exercise methods are good for building endurance and strength in the body, but they usually target specific muscle groups. In contrast, Yoga works the entire body simultaneously, creating harmony between the bones, muscles, and skin. This promotes freedom of movement, not only in the skeletal body, but also in the more subtle levels of energy, breath, and fluids. When our bodies are in harmony, we can turn off the stress response and begin lowering our cortisol and blood pressure.

Traditional exercise methods can also enervate rather than energize. Yoga, on the other hand, will never leave you feeling exhausted. In fact, it will leave you refreshed and even cheerful. I remember the days when I taught music in elementary school. I would come home wiped out and have to do a quick deep relaxation before I went off to teach my evening Yoga class. Once I got to class and did a few rounds of the sun salutation, though, I became completely refreshed and went home a new person.

We are multidimensional beings—intricate cohesions of body, mind, and spirit. The various practices of Yoga address all the facets of ourselves, bringing us into balance with a healthy body, a sharp mind, and an awareness of a deep abiding peace within. Additionally, many of Yoga's techniques and practices overlap and blend into each other. For instance, Hatha Yoga practice is primarily focused on the body, but because of its emphasis on the breath and inner awareness, it also becomes a meditation.

The medical community has been studying the health benefits of Yoga and has come up with several reasons why you might want to begin your practice today! One study found that a simple, daily meditation practice boosts the immune system, and the effects were evident long after the study was over. And that was just using meditation! Yoga's physical postures can rid your body of toxins, improve overall fitness, strengthen the cardiovascular system, balance organs and glands, and cure sleep and anxiety problems. Overall, the many benefits of Yoga, listed and discussed below, can easily improve the way you live your life.

Cleans out Toxins

If you've gotten discouraged with working out and have fallen off the exercise wagon, the reason could be that what you were doing wasn't working for you— either because it didn't feel good or wasn't fun. However, when we're inactive for awhile, toxins can build up in our bodies because the lymph system, which is like the "sewer" of the body, doesn't circulate. When this happens, it can make us feel bloated and tired. The lymph system doesn't have a pump like the circulatory system, so the only way lymph can move throughout the body is for *us* to move. As we come in and out of the Yoga postures, contracting and relaxing muscles, we are exerting gentle pressure on our organs. This helps to propel the lymph so it can remove toxins and fight infections.

Improves Overall Fitness

I know from my own personal struggles with weight, impulse control, and dietary indiscretions that I can slip into a downward spiral when I don't feel like exercising. Once I stop moving my body, it starts to murmur at me. "Oh, my hips are a little achy," or "Gee, my face looks puffy," and later, "Ouch! My back is killing me!" Pretty soon, all I want to do is sit on the couch and stare into space. So believe me, I've been there!

If you're feeling out of shape, you can improve your general fitness with Yoga. The obvious benefit is gaining flexibility, but you'd be surprised at how much it will improve your muscular strength and endurance, as well. It will even make your bones stronger. You can, and should start at your own pace. One of the key things that makes Yoga, Yoga, is that it allows us to relax our effort and come into poses that are steady and comfortable.

The standing poses are a good place to start developing strength and confidence. The tree pose, for example, focuses on balance and has the added benefit of improving concentration. In other standing poses, knee joints are nourished with fresh synovial fluid, which is squeezed into the cartilage and acts sort of like a shock absorber. Similarly, the health of the cartilage in spinal disks is improved in bending poses. These are things that can be measured, and the studies on Yoga have proven that it can be a key part of a healthy lifestyle.

Strengthens the Cardiovascular System

Some studies show that Yoga can minimize the negative health risks of being overweight. If you are carrying extra weight, you may have begun to experience some common health problems, which can be scary! And it doesn't help your blood pressure to be worrying about your blood pressure. *Big Yoga* actually focuses on some specific poses—especially the forward bends—that help to lower blood pressure and bring it back into normal range.

Additionally, regular Yoga practice can lower cholesterol and heart rate, as well as increase overall circulation—especially blood flow to the heart. The inverted poses allow the blood that's already been used up (spent, or venous blood) to flow back to the heart for recirculation. This helps reduce swollen ankles and gives the heart a little rest. In short, Yoga is heart healthy.

Balances Organs and Glands

All the stretching, twisting, and bending in Yoga provides a gentle massage to the internal organs and glands, helping to balance these delicate systems. For example, focusing attention on the breath during Yoga allows the lungs to expand and bring in more oxygen for greater vitality. The fish pose (Don't worry, all these poses and techniques will be discussed later in the book) opens the chest, which is especially beneficial to people with asthma. The side twists squeeze the pancreas and bring it a fresh supply of blood, which improves its function and stabilizes blood sugar; thereby reducing diabetics' need for insulin. Yoga also helps promote good bowel health, and backward bends help females alleviate menstrual problems and reduce female troubles. There have been studies that suggest a specific forward bend called the head-to-knee pose is beneficial to men's prostate health, as well.

The benefits do not end there. The thyroid gland, located at the base of the throat, gets stimulated during the shoulder stand. This helps to promote the production of thyroxin, the hormone that regulates metabolism. In addition, this pose drains the lymph system, promoting better immune function. I experienced this first-hand during my years teaching music in elementary schools. I avoided many colds and flus through my Yoga practice, and many of my clients have observed the same effect. It has even been shown that there is much less absenteeism—or just plain burnout—in the workplace when the employees are offered a noontime Yoga class.

Cures Sleep and Anxiety Problems

Some of my students complain that as they are getting older, they are having a harder time getting a good night's sleep. I, in turn, offer them a suggestion that worked for me when I was waking up at night, worrying about an ongoing legal situation. I advise them to do a gentle forward bend, knees slightly bent, head forward, breathing deeply and noisily at first, and gradually quieting and slowing the breath. I did this without even getting out of bed, and after about five minutes of this simple practice, I'd lie back down and fall fast asleep.

Another Yogic technique for calming the mind when it is agitated is chanting. You can begin chanting very loudly at the top of your voice and gradually get quieter. I like to use a chant taught by Swami Satchidananda. It goes, "*Hari Om, Hari Om, Hari Hari Hari Om.*" The Sanskrit word *Hari* is loosely translated to mean an aspect of God that removes obstacles. In combination with the universal mantra *om*, this little chant helps to engage the mind, but any short, uplifting chant will do. During chanting, the pineal gland—located in the center of the brain—is stimulated and releases melatonin, a hormone that is calming to the system. As your voice gets quieter, your mind will follow.

Another technique that helps bring about a peaceful night's sleep is a practice known as deep relaxation, or *Yoga Nidra*, which involves tensing and relaxing all the various parts of the body, followed by a soothing full body scan. In a Yoga class, deep relaxation happens toward the end—I like to think of it as the "dessert" of the class—and it is recommended by physicians as supporting and strengthening the cardiovascular system. Later in the book (page 194) there is a script you can use to talk yourself through this healing practice. In addition, you will learn how to soothe the brain with breathing exercises. By doing various breathing techniques, we balance the two hemispheres of the brain and re-oxygenate the blood. We also get into that yummy delta brain wave that is indicative of deep sleep.

Deep breathing, guided relaxation, and forward bends are just some of the ways we can bring the mind into stillness so that when our heads hit the pillows, we can sleep like babies, allowing our bodies to restore themselves. When we practice the various Yoga techniques, we become experts in controlling the stress response, so that we maintain our vitality and prevent disease.

THE HEALING POWER OF YOGA

Studies have shown that in addition to health benefits, Yoga actually has healing powers. It can restore to health people suffering from several conditions, because it teaches us how to handle stress. And stress is always a component in any bodily disease. The list of ailments Yoga can remedy goes on and on, and includes relief from ordinary problems like varicose veins, gas, PMS, constipation, and ADD. It is also helpful in more serious conditions, such as cancer and HIV.

Although certain Yoga poses can bring benefit to specific conditions, the best medicine for the body and mind is a sensible, easy practice of a variety of poses regularly. This will result in the gradual diminishing of little aches and pains. Even common maladies like backache, chronic fatigue syndrome, and carpal tunnel syndrome can be alleviated. Regular Yoga practice will result in your mind becoming sharp and your mood becoming joyous. You may even find you are experiencing a deeper spiritual connection.

The culmination of these benefits—and Yoga's greatest gift—is the sheer joy of being in a vibrant, healthy body, no matter its shape or size. You'll be amazed at how your body will respond, even after just one session. As an example, I had a student who was suffering from plantar fasciitis, a painful inflammation of the tendons of the feet. It was so painful that she had given up her morning jog and come to Yoga somewhat begrudgingly. At the end of class, however, she had a look on her face of sheer astonishment and disbelief. When she stood up to leave, she walked around the room testing her body out and said, "It feels so good to be able to walk again!" Yoga makes your body and mind feel better, which will make you feel better about everything!

Chapter 3

Beginning Your Yoga Practice

You now know quite a bit about Yoga and are probably anxious to get started. However, it's important to properly prepare yourself before doing so. Before your first Yoga session, you might want to check out some different Yoga videos from your local library and spend some time viewing them. They will give you an idea of what Yoga is all about and they can inspire you. Plus, you'll become familiar with some of the basic moves and terms, which will eventually become second nature to you. Don't think, however, that you have to look like the models in the videos. They are usually professionals who practice Yoga for several hours a day and have trained for years. If you find these models discouraging to watch, turn off the video! But remember, even these Yoga models had to start somewhere. And that's where you are now. Well, almost.

COMMON YOGA PROPS

For almost every form of exercise, it's best to have the right equipment and appropriate clothing. For instance, I recently wanted to go for a ride on my bike, but I realized I first needed a more comfortable seat and a new kickstand. Yoga is no exception. The nice thing about Yoga, though, is that you don't have to go overboard in order to do it right. Without having to make a major investment, you can prepare yourself for your first session. To start out, you can use simple household items, or you can go shopping! Let's look at some of the items you should have handy:

A Mat

You will want to perform your Yoga exercises on some type of mat. When I began studying Yoga, the ubiquitous sticky mat of today hadn't been invented! Instead,

23

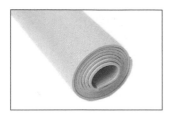

Sticky Mat

students were given large cotton towels, because cotton helps to wick away moisture from the body. Therefore, if you have a beach towel lying around the house, you can use it and it will work just fine. However, these days Yoga is most often done on mats made of rubber (recyclable) or PVC (not so much). These mats are sticky, which allows the feet to stick to the ground during the standing poses. They can be bought almost anywhere and can be doubled-up if you need extra cushioning under your knees or buttocks.

A Strap

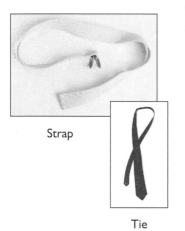

Strap

Tie

When the body is a little stiff, a canvas strap can be used to "lasso" a foot or hand in order to gently bring the body into position. These straps are available at Yoga studios, sporting goods stores, and even stores like Target and T.J. Maxx. Sometimes, you can get a kit that includes a sticky mat, a strap, and a video on how to use them. Another obvious resource is Amazon.com, and one of my students got her strap online from a website (probably Craigslist.com) where people give stuff away for free or sell it for cheap. Additionally, you can also use an old tie if you have one lying around. I actually picked up a bunch of ties at the local hand-me-down store for a buck each and they work just fine.

A Block

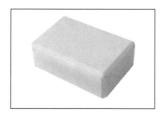

Block

Another popular Yoga prop is the block. Blocks give you support when you're stretching forward or sideways from a standing position and are unable to place your hands on the floor. They are typically made of cork or durable foam, and are available at sports stores, at your local Yoga studio, or online from any number of distributors of Yoga products. See the resource section (page 209) for some options. Or, try using a small cardboard box or even a nice fat book. Be creative!

A Blanket or Pillow

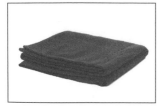

Blanket

When sitting cross-legged on the floor, it helps to have a folded blanket or pillow under the buttocks to raise it up, which allows the knees to relax and drop toward the floor. It also helps release tension in the groins. Again, you can use something you already have at home, or you can order a fancy one online. Blankets are available in wool, wool-blends, and cotton. Classic meditation pillows—sometimes referred to as a *zafus*—are usually round and have a strap for easy carrying. There are also newer versions that are crescent-shaped, as well as smaller, rectangular pillows. But don't forget, you also have pillows right there on your couch that might do the trick.

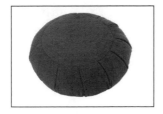

Zafu

A Sweater

At the end of my classes, I talk students through a deep relaxation that lasts anywhere from five to fifteen minutes. I recommend they bring an extra sweater to put on before we start so they don't get chilled. You should do the same. A large, soft pashmina works great and makes you feel pampered, too!

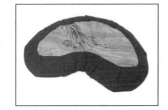

Crescent Pillow

An Outfit

Yoga clothing should be comfortable. Period. It shouldn't constrict you in any way or bind you at the waist. Some people feel most comfortable in a hoodie and sweats, and these days both items are available from many common stores (like J.C. Penney and Wal-Mart) in sizes up to 3 and 4X. Leotards, capris, and tights are also now available in larger sizes. (I know the Danskin brand offers these items up to 3 and 4X.) Personally, I like a little support in my Yoga duds, and usually wear something that is mostly cotton, with some lycra in it. Check the resources at the back of the book (page 212) for more information on plus-size activewear.

TIPS FOR MAXIMIZING THE BENEFITS
OF YOUR YOGA PRACTICE

In addition to gathering and/or purchasing props and clothing, there are a number of things you can do to prepare for your Yoga practice so that you get the most out of it. We all lead busy lives—getting kids off to school, shopping for groceries, organizing the recycling, getting to work, etc.—but Yoga can help us put it all in perspective. Here are some things you can do to maximize the benefits of your Yoga practice:

Practice on an Empty Stomach

Wait at least two to four hours after your last big meal and an hour or longer after a snack before practicing Yoga. This is because you want your body to assimilate all the benefits of your practice and not have energy drained away by the process of digestion. Also, you will be more comfortable if the stomach is empty. Additionally, I don't recommend drinking water during your practice, because it will cool down the internal process of burning toxins. And if you wait until after your session to have your water, it will help you shift your consciousness from a relaxed state to fully aware.

Shower

Come to your practice clean and empty. Try to have your morning elimination and shower before you begin. If you practice in the evening, a comfortable change of clothes and a quick wash of your face and hands should suffice. After all, Yoga is a sacred practice, and just like church or temple, you should clean yourself up before participating. In addition, your Yoga practice will cause you to sweat a little and eliminate toxins, so it's better to start out fresh.

Remove Jewelry and Other Restrictive Items

If you wear a watch, large earrings, necklaces, or any other jewelry items, be sure to remove them before you begin so they do not get in your way. Also, if you have long hair, have a scrunchy or rubber band nearby to tie it back during certain poses. And if your pants are a little tight around the waist, see if you can find something more stretchy.

Get Fresh Air

The room in which you practice Yoga should be warm and comfortable. But if it's not too cold or windy outside, open a window to let in some fresh air. Turn down any overhead lights, as well, and go for more ambient lighting to enhance the relaxing effect of the session. If you instead want to practice outside, that's great, but avoid doing so in direct sunlight during the heat of the day.

Move the Furniture

Make sure there's plenty of room for you to completely spread out and perform the poses. It's amazing how much space we take up when we allow ourselves to be open! So, move away any furniture that may get in your way before you begin.

Don't Use a Mirror

Do not scrutinize your every move in front of a mirror—at least not right away. Get in touch with your internal body first. Then, as you become more familiar with the poses, you can check your alignment in a mirror—especially if you are doing Yoga at home without an instructor.

Have a Special Yoga Mat

My teacher claimed that everything is alive with energy, and that by treating things with respect, we can raise vibrations to a higher level. For instance, did you know that love has a faster vibration than anger or hate? If this sounds like a lot of hooey to you, at least consider that when you use the same mat over and over, it begins to feel like home. It's less distracting because you have less to get accustomed to. You can feel that you are at home on your mat, even when you're in a Yoga studio with twenty other students. It's easy to settle down there, because you have settled down there before.

Set the Mood

Light a candle, offer some flowers, or put on some soft music to set a peaceful, relaxing mood. If you're into incense, light it about fifteen minutes before you begin so the air isn't too smoky, but you still feel its essence. If you choose to use music, keep the volume low and make sure it's not too engaging, or it will draw your awareness away from your practice.

Don't Wear Any Fragrances

Don't wear perfume, scented lotion, or anything else with a particularly fragrant scent—especially in public classes. This is in the category of good manners. Some people may be allergic to your perfume, fabric softener, or whatever it may be, and the smell will disturb their practice.

Alleviate Distractions

Keep your awareness within. If you're practicing at home, turn off the phone volume so you aren't listening to it ring, or to the answering machine as it's picking up your messages. If you're practicing in a Yoga studio, try not to compare yourself to anyone in the room—not even yourself. Yoga is not a competitive sport; rather, it's a method of transformation. If you try to match the expertise of your teacher or a fellow student, you may hurt yourself. The best way to avoid injury is to honor the body and pay attention to what it's feeling. This ability to observe the body will be enhanced over time, and you'll find yourself bringing consciousness to every part of the body.

Keep a Sturdy Chair Handy

If you find it difficult to get up and down from the floor, please use a chair to lean on for support. For coming up to a standing position from being on the mat, a sturdy child's chair is a good height. Additionally, a chair can be used in many of the poses' adaptations. In fact, the entire Yoga session can be performed using a chair, so it's a good idea to keep one close.

Keep the Breath Full and Relaxed

Yogic breathing brings energy to every part of the body. When there's more breath, there's more oxygen; more oxygen brings more prana (which we'll learn more about beginning on page 157); and more prana brings more joy and more aliveness. That's what it's all about! In Yoga, we always breathe through the nose with the mouth closed, unless otherwise indicated. The breath, though deep, is quiet—there should never be a sound of gasping or grunting—and is generally never held.

Exercise Caution
when Performing Inverted Poses

Inverted poses can be dangerous. Check with your doctor if you have retinal problems, glaucoma, migraines, high blood pressure, a hiatal hernia, or problems in the neck or head. Also, if you're nervous about performing a certain exercise like bringing your legs up the wall, ask a family member to spot you while doing your best to use your own muscles. Never fling yourself into a pose, though, because you could lose your balance and fall.

Avoid Inverted Poses during Menstruation

All poses during menstruation should be done especially gently, and women should refrain from practicing inverted poses when having their period. This is because inversion disrupts the body's natural, downward flow at this time of the month. Additionally, *Big Yoga* does not address the needs of pregnant women, who should never do any poses on their bellies after the first trimester. Therefore, please consult other sources suggested in the resource section (page 209) if you are pregnant. Know, though, that deep breathing can be very calming for you and the baby.

Shorten Your Practice if You're Pressured for Time

The most beneficial part of Yoga practice is the easiest part—the relaxation and breathing. So, if you only have time for one or two poses, simply do a short relaxation and some deep breathing. At least do a little of that everyday.

Gradually Build Your Routine

Slowly lengthen the time you hold each pose. You will notice I have given duration guidelines for both beginning and intermediate students throughout Part Two. Generally as a beginner, you should only hold the poses briefly, even for just a few breaths. If you want, you can do another repetition to build up strength, but please, don't strain! Over time, you'll naturally find yourself able and wanting to safely hold the poses longer.

A CAUTION OR TWO

The primary precaution I can offer you is to take it easy, especially as a beginning Yoga student. We Westerners are highly competitive, so it's not unusual for new students to overdo it in an effort to "get it right," to show off a little, or to "look like the picture." Trust me, though, it's not worth it. Respect your body at all times. Yoga is not a sport in which you should be trying to outdo your opponent—or yourself. For instance, you may find you're more flexible on one side than the other, or that today you can't stretch as far in a pose as you could yesterday. This is not unusual. It's fine to make these observations, but in Yoga we learn not to judge ourselves, or find ourselves lacking.

If you have health issues, such as high blood pressure, arthritis, any physical limitations because of your weight, or any lack of flexibility because of your age, please check with a medical professional that you trust before beginning Yoga. Additionally, throughout this book you'll see that I've provided you with a heads-up about cautions and considerations related to each pose depicted. However, with practice and dedication you will find that your body will actually begin to recover from physical ailments.

My teacher, Sri Swami Satchidananda, claimed that, "Health is your birthright!" Your beautiful body is designed to move, and Yoga practice will help you either maintain or regain an ease of movement that will give you a spring in your step, a smile on your face, and a twinkle in your eye. Soon, simple, everyday chores that may be a struggle for you now—like making the bed or getting in and out of the car—will become effortless.

YOGIC DIET

Swami Murugananda once said, "The road to health is paved with good *intestines*." Once you have made the decision to purify your system with Yoga, you should take some time to analyze your diet. Choose foods that make you healthy and calm. Become more mindful about what you put in your body, and eat life-giving foods—essentially, more veggies and less junk. Get local, organic produce whenever possible, and live by the simple idea of, "Whole foods, eaten whole."

The Yogic diet recommended by my teacher, Swami Satchidananda, was strictly vegetarian. Because it causes no harm to any sentient being, being a vegetarian puts you in alignment with a concept from the first limb of the tree of Yoga—the idea of *ahimsa,* or non-killing. My teacher Swamiji would give the example of animals in the zoo. The carnivores (meat-eaters), such as lions and tigers, are restless, pacing their cages. By contrast, the animals that are herbivores (plant-eaters), including the elephants, horses, and cows, are peaceful, but certainly not lacking in strength.

Swamiji also pointed out that the anatomy of herbivores is different from that of carnivores. Lions and tigers have big, sharp teeth made for tearing meat from the bone, and short digestive tracts to get the digested food out of the system before it putrefies. Have you ever given a hungry dog a bite of meat? He doesn't even chew it; he just gobbles it down! By comparison, goats, cows, and other grazing animals have flatter teeth made for chewing—like ours. And they have much longer digestive tracts—also like ours. Human intestines are thirty-three feet long! Grains take longer to break down than meat, and our longer digestive tracts enable our bodies to extract all the nutrients out of them.

Additionally, Dr. Dean Ornish, author of *Stress, Diet and Your Heart,* has shown the efficacy of a vegetarian diet through his success with patients suffering from heart disease. In his medical trials, which he based on the teachings of Swami Satchidananda, the patients were consistently able to reduce angina, lower cholesterol, and reduce plaque in the arteries—all by switching to a vegetarian diet and adding Yoga, light exercise, meditation, and group sharing to their routines. As a result, his patients were able to go home and live normal lives instead of having a costly bypass surgery.

Overall, the patients in Dr. Ornish's research reported a 91 percent average *reduction* in the frequency of chest pain due to heart disease. Back in 1977 when his research first began, the idea that coronary heart disease could be reversed was unheard of, but it quickly became hard to argue with Dr. Ornish's success. The lifestyle changes were something his patients could live with long-term, and most stayed in the program. When the participants were studied at the end of a five-year period, the progression of heart disease had stopped or begun to reverse itself in all but one person. And the more they continued to change their lifestyles, the better they felt and the more improvements they showed.

The Ornish program is not only medically effective, but it is also cost effective. According to Dr. Ornish's book, every patient who chooses to try his program's lifestyle changes rather than opt for bypass surgery, saves approximately $50,500. And that is just the monetary savings! It doesn't take into account the pain and trauma avoided by not undergoing any surgery.

Personally, I follow a vegetarian diet, but if that seems too limiting for you, simply try to incorporate more and more plant-based foods into your diet. It took me a few years of modifying my diet before I became a complete vegetarian. Then, during my menopause years, I fell back into eating meat as a way of curbing intense cravings brought about by my shifting hormones. Today, I am once again a happy vegetarian, and I recommend it to anyone who is serious about Yoga. The best way to learn how to eliminate meat from your diet is to hang out with other vegetarians, but if you have questions about switching to a vegetarian diet, make sure you check with a nutritionist or read up on the subject to inform yourself. Food can be healthful and delicious. Sometimes it can be eaten in celebration, other times it may be eaten simply to get the job done. But it should never be a punishment or a source of shame.

CHECK SELF-LOATHING AT THE DOOR

I have never had a student that didn't have some body issues, no matter how thin, young, or beautiful they were. So don't be surprised if, or should I say, when, your mind starts telling you all the reasons why you can't do Yoga. It may be that you have reservations about your ability to do some of the poses found in this book. But don't let that stop you! It is not essential to achieve a certain level of proficiency to receive benefit from the poses.

Regardless of your ability level, bring yourself to this ancient practice and listen to your body. Stretch to the edge of your comfort zone and rest there, with conscious attention to the breath. Try to have a short deep relaxation after your Hatha practice, and even a little deep breathing. Then, you will naturally have a beautiful moment of stillness, and I won't have to tell you the delicious feeling that will bring. Like the experience of eating a juicy, ripe peach, the benefits of Yoga cannot be described. You have to taste it for yourself.

In addition to physical reservations, you may feel you have some bad habits that are keeping you from doing Yoga. You might think you need to give up smoking, drinking, overeating, purging, or whatever you label as "bad," before you begin your Yoga practice. While eliminating unhealthy habits is something we all strive for, don't put off doing Yoga because you feel you're not ready. Go ahead and introduce it into your life, and gradually you will develop such a love for your new, "good" habit that you won't feel so eager to indulge in your old ways. And as part of your Yoga practice, you should begin to neutralize the judgments you make about your behaviors. You are exactly as God intended you to be.

Chapter 4

Overcoming Stumbling Blocks

If done regularly, Yoga can have a cumulative effect on the body and mind, and the results can change your health and well-being for the better. Too often, though, excuses get in the way of this ultimate achievement. We all have our own reasons for not getting on the Yoga mat on any given day. I've been practicing Yoga for over thirty years and I still have a worldbook full of excuses!

Some days, I simply act as if I want to do my exercises. Acting "as if" is a very useful tool in making positive changes in our lives. William James, the father of American psychology, was credited with coming up with the idea. He claimed, "If you want a quality, act 'as if' you already had it." When you do this, a part of your brain known as the Reticular Activating System (RAS) directs your behavior to narrow the gap between where you are in consciousness, and where you want to be. In my case, when I need to do my Yoga even when I'm not feeling it, I'll just take some action, like putting on my sweatpants or sitting on

> "The energy of the universe is yours. It is your birthright. Just claim it."
> YOGI BHAJAN

my meditation pillow. Then, I find myself moving to my mat, and once there, I fall into a comforting routine and am glad I did. This chapter is comprised of several common excuses people use to avoid Yoga, followed by tricks to transcend them. Some of them just might sound familiar to you!

I DON'T HAVE ENOUGH TIME

I think this one is true for all of us! Our culture has scheduled itself into oblivion. All of us, including our children, are constantly trying to beat the clock, and are beating ourselves up in the process! If, like most people these days, you are juggling a career, a family, church or temple, community sevice, excercise, and aspirations for a spiritual life, you may find your needs are at the bottom of the deck.

However, the next time you are feeling overwhelmed and pressured for time, remind yourself that you can still squeeze in some Yoga. You don't have to do every pose, everytime to make it count. It's much better to do a simple, short practice regularly than it is to do a long, intense practice only once or twice a month. You also may find you prefer certain poses more than others. That's fine. All that means is that your inner *guru,* or teacher, is helping you discover what you need.

Finally, I know it sounds a little farfetched, but regular Yoga practice can actually make time seemingly expand by improving your physical and mental capabilities and awareness. Yoga's physical poses are designed to squeeze toxins out of the body's soft tissues and give a nice massage to the internal organs, tuning them up to work more effectively. In addition, the meditation involved in Yoga is intended to sharpen your mind, and deep Yogic breathing is an excellent way to bring more energy into the body, giving you better endurance and better immunity to diseases. With a well-tuned body, keen mind, and improved energy and endurance, you will begin each day at the top of your game. Solutions to problems will become more obvious, and the length of time it takes you to perform various activities will be reduced. In short, you will feel like you have more time.

I DON'T HAVE A PLACE TO DO YOGA

So, make one! It isn't a myth that Yoga practice is helped when it is performed in a sacred space. After all, don't candles, bubble bath, and bathtub pillows help us relax more and luxuriate in the tub? With that same frame of mind, creating a niche in our homes that has at least some of the elements of an alter can help us peacefully practice Yoga. At the very least, have a special candle that you only light during meditation and Hatha Yoga practice. The candle will help you remember that you are light.

Besides a candle, you may also want to offer some flowers and have a visual image of a saintly person in your special Yoga space. For instance, when my children were little I often kept a picture of Mother Mary on my altar, to inspire me to be a good mother. Your neighborhood Yoga studio or New Age bookstore will have pictures, statues, and religious art of a wide variety of faiths, so go check them out and find one that speaks to you. Lord Buddha once said, "As we think, so we become." By meditating on a person who inspires you, you may begin to take on some of his or her supreme qualities.

Another nice addition to an altar is a concentric geometric pattern called a *mandala*—also refered to as a *yantra. Mandala* is a combination of two ancient Sanskrit words, meaning "having" and "essence." Mandalas and yantras are visual representations of a sacred sound, such as "om," or symbolic depictions of the cosmos themselves. In the center of the diagram there is often a red dot called a *bindu,* and by gazing at it, we experience the holy vibration of that sound at a very subtle level. Or, we may even experience a feeling of oneness with the entire cosmos!

Additionally, you might consider having some Mala beads on hand. Mala beads are prayer bead necklaces made of 108 beads plus a center bead, or *mehru.* They come in all types—from humble sandalwood to precious stones like citrine, amethyst, and crystal. Originally from the Middle East, Mala beads evolved into the Western rosary after the crusaders observed the Muslims praying with their prayer beads. They then brought the idea back to the West. The reason prayer beads and rosaries are used in so many diverse traditions is because they are effective in keeping the mind focused on the mantra. After each mantra repetition, for instance, "All is One," or "Om Shanthi," you move on to the next bead until you come to the *mehru.* Then, simply turn the beads around and continue for as long as you like.

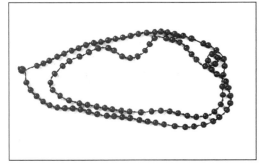

Mala Beads

Finally, in your Yoga space you should keep a sticky mat, special rug, or even a towel that is used only for your Hatha practice. Make sure it is in a place where it won't get trampled on. Objects carry vibrations, and by treating your meditation objects with respect, you will make them sacred.

IT'S TOO NOISY WHERE I LIVE

For me, noise can be a distraction from my Yoga practice. For instance, in the afternoons, instead of meditating on my inner peace, I sometimes find myself meditating on the neighbor's barking dog or leaf blower. So, I've found that the best time for me to meditate is before six in the morning, when the world is sleeping peacefully. Swami Sivananda, the great sage of Rishikesh and my teacher's Guru, actually said that we should be "up and doing" at four in the morning, because the vibrations at that hour are more conducive to meditation.

If you simply can't get up that early, though, and the noises of the day have already begun, try putting on a CD of peaceful meditative music. It can help block out the noise from the street, and yet, not be too distracting. In fact, Swamiji, my beloved teacher, once suggested that I create a meditation CD. I named it "Omniscient Om" and used the repetion of "om" over a background of piano improvisation. Now, every time I put it on, it envelops me in a bubble of peaceful vibrations. I also like to listen to ambient music that is not very melodic and a little mind-numbing. I am a big fan of Harold Budd and Brian Eno. Check out the resource section (page 209) for more suggestions.

MY KIDS COME IN WHEN I'M TRYING TO DO YOGA

That's great! You can begin to teach them Yoga, too! It's really important to give children an opportunity to experience a peaceful state. Their worlds are full of commotion, hurry, and noise (not that yours isn't!), and by giving them a simple Yoga practice all their own you will be doing both you and them a big favor. Even by teaching them simple breathing exercises, you will be giving them life-long tools for relaxation.

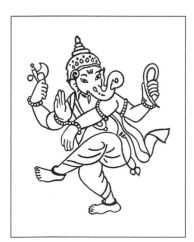

Sanskrit "Om"

If that doesn't work, try a different approach. Most kids love to play with fire and smoke, so give them a stick of incense that they can gently wave at your Yoga candle. Teach them to draw the letters "O" and "M" in the air with it, or teach them the Sanskrit symbol for "om." When they're a little older, they can even be the one to light your Yoga candle.

Another option you have is to let your children make up their own prayers. It's okay to play with God! Those of us who grew up in the Judea-Christian tradition are accustomed to thinking that there is only one God, but in the Eastern religions, there can be many names and forms of God. For instance, one of the things I love about the Hindu tradition is the way they see God in everything! Your kids will love the colorful stories about the different Hindu gods—actually they are various aspects of the One God—such as Lord Ganesha, who has the body of a man, and the head of an elephant! Or, Hanuman, the monkey god who is known for his great strength. Or Lord Nataraj, who is half man, half woman, and dances in a ring of fire!

When my kids used to come in and pester me while I was doing Yoga, I would start teaching them some poses and they'd almost immediately get bored and go away. Other mothers have told me they keep a special Yoga toy basket full of quiet activities to be used just during mommy's Yoga time. Figure out what works for your family,

Lord Ganesha

and begin enjoying Yoga with your children.

I'M TOO STIFF

If you are a normal, everyday American who eats at fast food restuarants, goes everywhere by car, smokes cigarettes (or worse), or drinks alcohol frequently, you may not be feeling so great. This is probably an exaggeration on reality, but lack of exercise, a toxic diet, and a fast-paced lifestyle can create stresses that manifest as a stiff, achy body and a cranky mind. But don't let this put you off your Yoga practice, and don't use it as an excuse! The physical poses will help to squeeze the toxins—the primary source of the stiffness—out of the body and loosen things up. In addition, the breathing practices will help to purify the blood, removing toxins at a more subtle level.

You have to start somewhere. If you're stiff, so be it. Part of Yoga is to accept your body as it is and love it anyway. The body has amazing healing capabilities, and regular Yoga practice can ignite and accelerate them. A.E. Alexander, creator of the Alexander Technique (a movement therapy that helps the student become aware of painful, unconscious postural habits), uses a term that I love to describe this healing power. He calls it the "righting reflex." It means that, given the proper opportunity, the body has a natural ability to correct itself. And with just a little effort, the body will start to come around. So, have faith. The ancient Vedic scriptures purport, *"Mana eva manushyanam karanam bandhamokshayoh."* ("If you think you are bound, you are bound. If you think you are free, you are free.")

I CAN'T FIND
YOGA CLOTHING IN MY SIZE

Some of the greatest benefits of writing this book were the wonderful resources and information I came across during my research. I have found so many things online that I never knew existed! For instance, did you know there is an entire movement afoot called Fat Acceptance? Or that there is a website called www.PlusSizeYellow-Pages.com? If you have access to a computer—go to the library if you're desperate—you can easily go online and find everything you need for your Yoga practice, regardless of your size. Junonia and Always for Me.com's online catalogs are a good place to start, especially for Yoga togs. There is a list of several cool websites that carry plus-size activewear in the resource section at the back of the book (page 212).

I HAVE HEALTH ISSUES

Many people new to Yoga have some health issues. Maybe yours are even the reason why you picked up this book in the first place. In a way, though, pain and ill health can be your friends if they are what ultimately convince you to take action and and begin to better care for yourself. You can either let your maladies rule your life, or you can take control of them. Yoga is a gentle and effective way to begin improving your physical and mental well-being. So, congratulations to you for taking the first step!

Most health problems will not prevent you from doing an easy Yoga practice, so no more excuses. Whether you're stiff from arthritis, on medication for high blood pressure, on insulin for diabetes, or have other challenges, you still can find your way to the mat or chair for a regular Yoga session. (If you're recovering from surgery, check with your doctor to make sure your stiches have healed completely and it's okay to do Yoga.) Maybe your practice won't look like pictures of Yoga that you've seen in magazines—I wouldn't recommend standing on your head, for instance!—but it will still be beneficial. And over time, you will begin to notice your conditions improving.

> *"Take it easy, not lazy."*
> Swami Satchidananda

The Hatha poses in *Big Yoga* are designed to provide bigger bodies a gentle toning of the glands, organs, and nerves, as well as to promote greater flexibility. When you combine exercises from different categories (warm-ups, forward bends, backward bends, etc.), your body will get a complete tune-up and will thank you. Before you perform any pose pictured in the book, though, make sure you read its complete description. Included in each is a consideration section, where you can check to see if your particular health issue is mentioned. Check in with yourself, as well. No one knows your body as well as you do.

A Word about High Blood Pressure

There are certain poses that are not recommended for people with high blood pressure, particularly the inversions. However, if you're taking your medication and get your doctor's approval, most of the poses in this book can be done even with this condition. Be sure to check each description and fully read the considerations, though, so you'll know which poses to avoid or modify. Then, if you begin a regular Yoga practice, your blood pressure may go down and stay down, allowing you to incorporate those poses into your routine.

I CAN'T AFFORD TO GO TO A REGULAR CLASS

These days, Yoga is a big business and the cost of attending classes can quickly add up—especially if you're a beginner and really want to immerse yourself in learning. Sometimes, Yoga studios will give you a good deal if you buy a month's worth of classes, so be sure to ask around. Signing up for a plan like that is also a good incentive to keep up your practice. Additionally, if you aren't employed full time, you might offer *seva*, or service, to the the studio in exchange for classes.

Although there really isn't any substitute for having an inspired teacher, sometimes it just isn't practical. If that is the case, go out and buy a new or used Yoga DVD, or borrow one from your local library. Then, watch and study it a few times before actually practicing. This may sound silly, but you will get some benefits simply through observation! Once you feel you have the hang of the poses, try doing the class along with the video. After awhile you won't even need to look at the TV, you will will be able to just listen, draw your awareness within, and have a beautiful, meditative experience.

If possible, supplement your at-home Yoga practice with an occassional group class at your local YMCA or Park and Recreation Center. If they don't offer Yoga classes in your community, ask for them! There are lots of Yoga teachers around these days, and they need you as much as you need them. The bottom line is that, regardless of your budget, there are ways to attend real or virtual classes.

I'M INVOLVED IN A FIGHT

At certain points in all of our lives, we get caught in emotional webs of anger and resentment and can't seem to find our way out. Or, we find ourselves with hurt feelings because someone treated us unkindly. Harboring negative emotions can make it hard to settle down and practice Yoga. So, what can we do with these overpowering emotions? Thankfully, the Yogis have thought of everything. In Patanjali's *Yoga Sutras*, he very briefly discusses how to calm the mind when it's churning with emotion. Book 1, Sutra 33, states: "By cultivating attitudes of friendliness to the happy, compassion toward the unhappy, delight in the virtuous, and disregard for the wicked, the mindstuff retains its undisturbed calmness." (Translation by Sri Swami Satchidananda in his book *The Yoga Sutras of Patanjali*, used with permission.)

Because the sutras are very brief, that's really all Patanjali had to say. But Swami Satchidananda elaborated on his basic message, and called these attitudes the four locks and the four keys. Any time you come across a "lock," apply the proper "key" and you can keep your mind calm. In other words, when you meet a happy person, what's the best way to act? Jealous? No. Simply be friendly and enjoy his or her happiness. There's no need to try to bring a happy person down if you're feeling low yourself. And what about meeting an unhappy person? Does Patanjali suggest you try to offer him or her advice or cheer? No. Simply have compassion. If there's something that unhappy person asks you for and you can give it, that's okay, too. But there's no suggestion that you have to "fix" him or her.

If you're fortunate enough to meet a truly virtuous person, just delight in his or her presence and maybe try to cultivate the virtuous qualities that you admire most. Remember, the whole point of the four locks and the four keys is to keep the mind calm. And finally, what about that terrible, wicked, (annoying, stupid, fill in your own adjective) person who makes your blood boil? This is the real challenge. Do your best to simply disregard him or her. Although it's not as easy as it sounds, it's a profound practice for strengthening the mind. A beautiful technique that helps us in this fourth key is the practice of *Pratipaksha Bhavana*, in which we replace a negative thought with a positive one. You don't have to like everybody when you're a Yogi, but you can have compassion for even those who treat you badly. That being said, there's nothing wrong with staying away from bad people. You are like a tender young tree—it is helpful to put up a fence around it until it becomes a sturdy oak.

I have found these locks and keys to be a great comfort during stressful times, although they can apply to almost any situation. Often by simply meditating on my problems with compassion and equanimity, the solutions present themselves effortlessly. So, instead of avoiding Yoga when you're upset, flock to it! It will help you sort out your emotions and clear your mind.

I'D RATHER GO TO THE MOVIES

My teacher, Swami Satchidananda, often spoke about perfection in action. What is a perfect act? He described it as one that harms no one and helps someone—even if that someone is just yourself. So, in deciding your priorities, think about what an action's benefits are, as well as who will likely receive those benefits. Will you get more benefit from the movies (which can be great stress busters, especially if they're funny and get you laughing), or from Yoga class? Will it hurt anyone if you go to the movies? Who needs your entrance fee more—the Yoga studio or the movie theater? Always take time to analyze your motives. And whether you realize it or not, this, too, is Yoga.

I DON'T FEEL COMFORTABLE IN YOGA CLASS

The ability to comfortably attend class with a Yoga teacher you trust is important, so take control of your own situation. Begin by finding a beginners class in your area. Get to your first class early and meet privately with the teacher before it starts. Ask about his or her experience with adapting poses for larger bodies and try to get a feel for the situation. See if the approach used seems expansive, or if you feel the teacher wants to jam you into some pre-conceived ideas of how Yoga should look. If you get a funny vibe and it doesn't feel right, follow your instincts and keep looking.

If, however, you feel comfortable enough with the instructor after your meeting, go ahead and take the class. Sometimes, Yoga teachers get a little overzealous and want to "help" students get deeper into poses, so be sure to let yours know at the beginning of class whether or not you want to be touched. Personally, I prefer to give my students verbal cues, and allow them to explore each pose in their own unique ways. And if you're ever stuggling during class, don't hesitate to raise your hand and ask for a quiet consultation.

> *"When the student is ready, the teacher appears."*
> BUDDHIST PROVERB

Finally, why not consider becoming a Yoga teacher yourself? There are currently over 18,000 people teaching Yoga in the United States, but how many of them are teaching *Big Yoga*? Look for teacher trainings in your area. Many large Yoga studios offer teacher trainings. You can also go online, check in Yoga magazines, or even contact me. If you can learn to share the gift of *Big Yoga*, you will not only be providing a wonderful service to others, you will deepen your own practice, as well.

STAY STRONG!

It's pretty much a guarantee that anytime we resolve to start a new fitness routine or diet, or to make a lifestyle change, we will be met with resistance. It sometimes seems like it's one step forward, two steps back. But through it all, have patience with yourself and don't give up. You'll receive so much benefit from doing Yoga at least a few times a week, that it's worth it to press through your lethargic tendencies. And as I mentioned earlier, you don't have to do every pose everyday!

In fact, it's a good idea to alternate between different routines so you don't get bored. Take some time and determine what works best for you. For instance, instead of doing your Yoga practice on your own, you might prefer teaming up with a friend or neighbor so you can encourage each other. Or, if you find you're not regular with your at-home practice, you might be better off signing up for classes at your local Yoga studio or community recreation center. If you have a little extra cash, see what DVDs are available online, but don't blow a lot of money all at once. I think I'm safe in saying that we have all made the mistake of buying exercise videos when we're on a self-improvement kick, only to find them sitting in the cupboard, unopened and unused, a month or so later.

Personally, I find that when I really need a Yoga tune-up I receive the most inspiration from spending time at a Yoga ashram. It's like Yoga camp! Many contemporary ashrams offer weekend retreats, month-long teacher trainings, and private retreats for various lengths of time. At ashrams, there are usually regularly scheduled meditations, Hatha classes, delicious vegetarian meals, and chanting sessions. Also, they offer a place to socialize with other Yoga students and teachers, and build supportive relationships. You can find a list of Yoga ashrams in the resource section at the back of the book (page 211).

There are times and circumstances in all of our lives that warrant, and sometimes require, change. When those occur, it's important that we stick to our goals so we don't get frustrated and end up throwing in the towel. Set aside the time to make Yoga part of your lifestyle. After awhile, the day may even come where you really miss your Yoga if you don't do it! Ultimately, Yoga is about disciplining your mind and body to achieve the greater goal of feeling peaceful, easeful, and useful—not just on the mat, but all throughout your life.

LET'S GET STARTED!

Hopefully, you now have your mat, block, pillows, and other goodies, and have carved out an hour or so in your busy life to take good care of yourself. You may have even viewed a couple of Yoga DVDs from the library or borrowed one from a friend, and heard the names of the poses—salute to the sun, downward dog, and child's pose to name a few—enough times so that you have a sense of what they are and how they look.

However, in Part Two of this book you'll see a different kind of Yoga model: Me, a "Big Yogi." (The word *Yogi* is a shortened version of the ancient Sanskrit word *Yogin,* generally denoting a male Yogi. The feminine is *Yogini.* In the interest of gender neutrality and ease of use, however, I am using Yogi throughout this book to mean both men and women who practice Yoga.) I'll show you how the poses look when they're being performed by a bodacious, curvy girl. I'll be demonstrating the traditional pose, and then offering adaptations that might be helpful for you depending on where you are stiff and where you carry your weight. Remember—you don't have to be thin to enjoy the benefits of Yoga. Now, let's get started!

Part Two

Yoga Practices

This part of the book contains descriptions and photographs of Yoga's physical poses. Because of the limitless variations of human bodies, there are as many adaptations of the classical Yoga postures as there are stars in the infinite sky. Thus, even within the narrow niche of *Big Yoga*, we still can come up with hundreds—maybe thousands—of versions of the poses, several of which are included in this book. How you should perform the different postures all depends on where you carry your weight, where you have stiffness or injury, whether you're a newbie or an experienced Yogi, and how committed you are to a regular practice. Just remember that this is *your* Yoga. The pictures of the poses in the following chapters show how *my* body does Yoga, but they will provide you with a good jumping off point for you to explore how your own body performs.

The first chapter in this part includes sections that describe and depict warm-ups and resting poses, backward bends, forward bends, inversions, twists, standing poses, and seated poses. What follows is a chapter that discusses the benefits of breath, as well as lays out several different breathing techniques. Next, we will learn about the powerful effects of meditation. And finally, we conclude with Yoga's service and devotional aspects.

In sequencing your Yoga session, it is helpful to set up a program that follows the order of the sections as they appear in this book. In other words, begin with the warm-ups and continue through to the seated poses. You don't have to do each pose in each section. Just choose one or two and then move on. Be sure to leave a little time at the end of your practice for a short, deep relaxation and a few of the breathing exercises, and you'll be good to go. In Integral Yoga, on which *Big Yoga* is based, it's important to include these last two items with each session, as it's the time when the body has a chance to right itself. So, manage your time well and do your best to include these profound practices as part of all of your Yoga sessions.

As a final note, when you approach these postures, be kind to your body and don't ever force anything. Anytime you begin to feel uncomfortable in a pose, back off a little until you feel the body release the tension. You'll get the maximum benefit from your Yoga by staying relaxed in every pose, so find the sweet spot where you're feeling invigorated without strain. With that being said, it's time to begin your own Yogic journey. Good luck and enjoy!

Chapter 5

Hatha Yoga Poses

Now that we have learned about the evolution of Yoga and Yoga's benefits, as well as what we need to get started and solutions for overcoming stumbling blocks, it's time to dive into the Hatha Yoga poses! Be sure to read through the benefits of each pose, so you come to realize all of the wonderful things you are doing for your body.

We will begin by going through various warm-ups, which bring fresh blood and energy to the muscles and joints, and literally warm them up, thereby preventing injury. Also included in the warm-up section are resting poses, which provide a way to keep your practice calm and centered. When we train the body to rest, we can rebound from stressful situations more quickly.

After our warm-ups, we move into backward bends, which tone the muscles that support the spine, keeping it supple and young. Backward bends should always be paired with forward bends to keep the body balanced, so naturally, a section on forward bends follows. In the forward bends, we begin to become aware of the calming effects of the Yoga poses.

Next are the inversions, and you'll definitely want to try them! Try to recollect the image of a child's delight when being held upside down by a loving parent—it feels great! Then, we look at the twists. Twists give the spine a nice wringing out, and they also subtly tone the organs and glands. For strength and balance, we offer standing poses. And finally, we offer several seated poses for meditation and digestive health. As one last reminder, it's best to set up your practice in the same order as the following sections appear, interjecting the standing and seated poses whenever necessary.

Warm-Ups

There's nothing more demoralizing than vigorously starting out a new exercise program, only to wind up out of commission because you've hurt yourself! In Yoga, as with any physical exercise, it's important to warm up the body before going onto the more strenuous poses. Warming up properly will help you avoid injury.

Many of the following warm-up exercises help to lubricate the muscles and joints by bringing more blood and synovial fluid to them. This gentle lubrication can even be healing in its own right! Other poses described in this section are transitions, which allow the body to rest and rebalance between different poses. If you're new to Yoga, you might want to take some time practicing just these exercises for the first week or two, to tone and strengthen your muscles. You'll be amazed at how great these basic warm-ups can make you feel!

1. Eye Exercises
   Nethra Viyaayaamam

5. Reclining Buddha
   Sayana Buddhasana

2. Salute to the Sun
   Soorya Namaskaaram

6. Cat Pose
   Biralasana

3. Supine Corpse
   Savaasana

7. Happy Baby
   Prasanna Shishu

4. Prone Corpse
   Advaasana

8. Rock the Baby
   Dolaayaate Shishu

1. Eye Exercises
Nethra Viyaayaamam

BENEFIT

Eye exercises strengthen and tone the eyes, and also increase blood flow to the optic nerve. Because the optic nerve is a part of the brain, these eye movements help to improve concentration, making them ideal for the beginning of each Yoga session, or before meditation.

TECHNIQUE

Sitting in comfortable position—either crossed legged on the floor, or on a chair with the feet on the floor—close the eyes and begin watching the breath. Feel the spine getting long and the shoulders wide. Keep the neck soft and the head still throughout the eye movements. With all of the following eye exercises, begin slowly and gradually increase the speed of the movements. After each exercise, close the eyes and let them go soft.

DURATION

Beginner: Three or four repetitions of each exercise, performed consecutively, are recommended.

Intermediate: After several weeks of practice, you can jump right to the circular movements. Three rounds in each direction should be sufficient, but up to fifteen repetitions are recommended by my teacher, Swami Satchidananda.

CONSIDERATION

Give the eyes a good stretch as you would any muscle. The emphasis is on the stretching rather than the seeing—in other words, don't worry about focusing on anything in front of you. Be careful not to strain the eyes. If you feel any discomfort, such as tightness, burning, or sharp or dull pains, close the eyes and place the palms over them for a minute until the discomfort subsides, and discontinue the eye exercises until the following Yoga session.

Exercise 1. Horizontal Movements

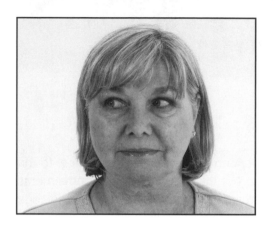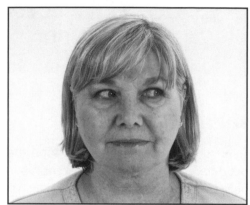

Open the eyes and look to the right. Then, come across the vision in a straight line to the left, keeping the movements fluid. Bring the eyes back to center before closing and relaxing them.

Exercise 2. Vertical Movements

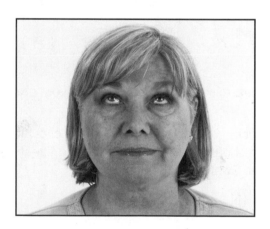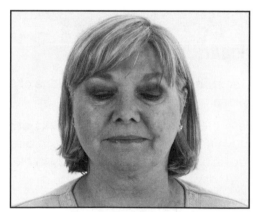

Open the eyes and look up. Glide the eyes downward in a straight line as far as you can without straining, remembering to keep the head still. Bring the eyes back to center, and then close and relax them.

Exercise 3. Diagonal Movements

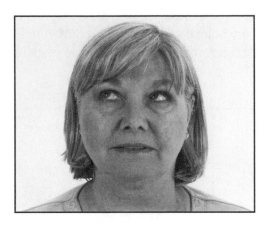 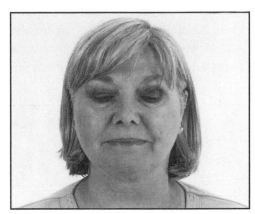

Move the eyes from the upper right corner of the vision to the lower left corner, then back up to the right. If you have difficulty keeping the line straight, hold your index finger out in front of you and use it to trace a diagonal line for your eyes to follow. Trace the diagonal in each direction a few times, and then bring the eyes to center to close and relax them.

Exercise 4. Opposite Diagonal Movements

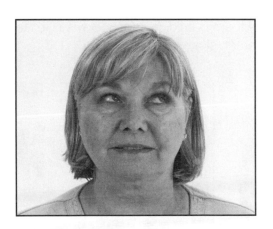 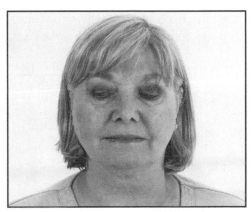

Opening the eyes once again, look up to the left corner of the vision then bring the eyes down to the right, trying to draw a straight line. After a few rounds, center the eyes and close, relaxing them thoroughly.

Exercise 5. Clockwise Circular Movements

Imagine the face of a clock and open the eyes to look at the twelve. Then, make clockwise circles with your eyes, touching every point on the circle's circumference. Start slowly, then pick up the pace a bit. After a few rounds, bring the eyes back to center and close them, letting them go soft.

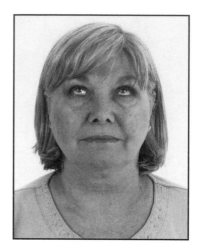 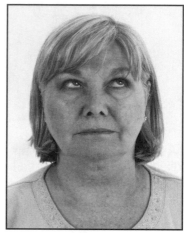 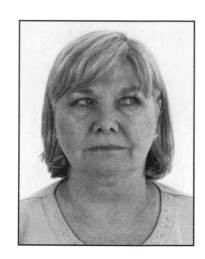

Exercise 6. Counter-Clockwise Circular Movements

Open the eyes and look upward. Then, move them in fluid counterclockwise circles for a few rotations. Bring the eyes back to center, close, and relax them.

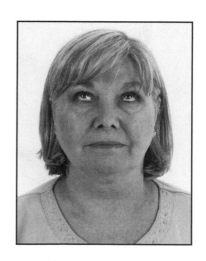 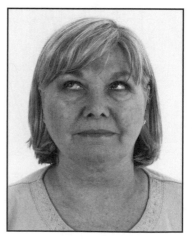 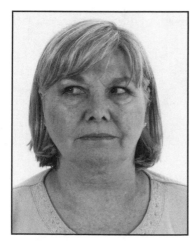

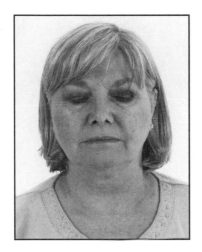
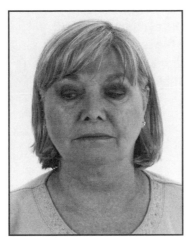
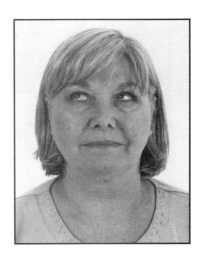

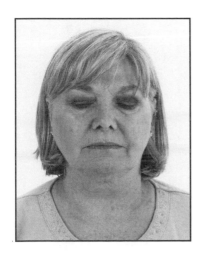
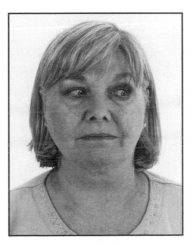
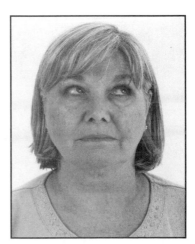

Recovery

With the eyes closed, briskly rub the palms of the hands together to generate some heat. Cup the warm palms over the closed eyes, and let them be soothed by the energy and warmth in the palms. When the heat subsides, bring the fingertips down to the closed eyes and massage gently out toward the temples a few times. Finally, bring the hands to the lap and take a moment to feel the soft feeling in the eyes.

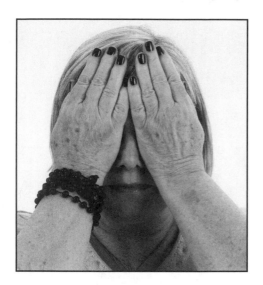

2. Salute to the Sun
Soorya Namaskaaram

BENEFIT

The sun salutation is a wonderful tonic for the whole body. When you're feeling a little sluggish or sleepy, you can do it rapidly to wake and revitalize the body. Conversely, you can also do it slowly and prayerfully to quiet the restless mind.

TECHNIQUE

The traditional sun salutation is a dynamic series of twelve poses that flow from one into the next. They help limber up the body for the rest of the Yoga session. When performed on the floor, the sun salutation can be challenging for the Big Yogi. Therefore, the following is a wall adaptation of the traditional floor exercise, which gives the same benefits without causing undue strain.

DURATION

Beginner: It isn't necessary to hold each position. Simply go at your own pace and create a graceful flow. Three repetitions of all twelve positions are good for beginners.

Intermediate: When you are able to do three rounds comfortably, try building up to nine repetitions over time. Done rapidly, this is a good fat-burner!

CONSIDERATION

Do not overexert! When coming up out of the standing forward bend, be especially careful not to hold the breath or strain. If you have any retinal problems, be careful to observe any increase in the pressure in the head. Go at your own pace, in a loving way. If you need extra support, walk the hands up and down the wall. Or, try the adaptation provided, which uses a chair.

"If you lean against a wall, it helps you. If you bang your head against it, it hurts you. You get a reward or punishment according to your approach. You are the cause of it all."
SWAMI SATCHIDANANDA

Position 1

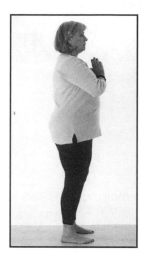

Facing a wall, stand with the feet parallel and bring the palms together under the chin. Feel yourself grounded to the earth, with the top of the head lifting toward the sky.

Position 2

a. Inhale and sweep the arms out to the sides.

b. Continue to breathe as you bring both arms overhead.

c. Clasp the hands together above the head and exhale as you stretch gently backwards.

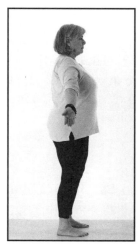
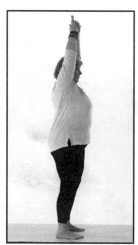
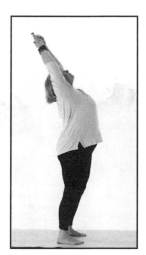

Position 3

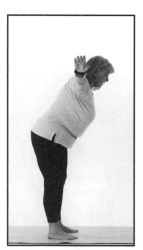

Stretch up again on an inhale. Then, separate the arms and make a "swan dive" down, bending at the hips like a hinge until the arms are hanging loosely toward the floor.

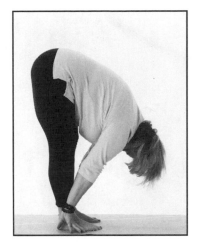

Position 4

With the legs straight or slightly bent, let the arms dangle and allow the weight of the arms and head draw the body down.

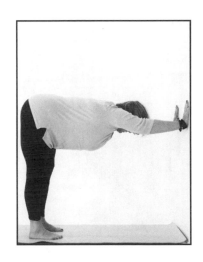

Position 5

Coming into what is called the wall dog, inhale and place the palms flat against the wall at hip-level. You can walk them up the wall for support if you need to. Keep the back, arms, and legs long, and the chest open. The arms are alongside the ears, and the face is looking toward the floor. This is an adapted version of the traditional downward dog pose (page 100).

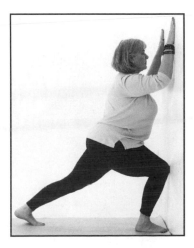

Position 6

Inhale as you bring the right foot forward to the wall, leaving the left foot in place but allowing the heel to come up off the floor. Bend the right knee, coming into a lunge position, as you stretch the arms up the wall as far as you are comfortable. The forearms will be parallel to the wall, almost touching it. Look toward the wall, softening the back of the neck. Breathe deeply, bringing awareness to the rib-cage.

Position 7

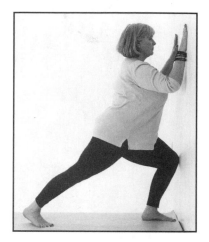

Bring the palms down the wall slightly as you switch the legs, bringing the right leg back and the left leg forward to the wall into the lunge. You can allow the wall to support the forward knee, and you can even let the chest rest on the wall. Adjust the palms up the wall, just above the shoulders, and look straight forward. Breathe deeply, feeling the lungs fill up along the side ribs.

Position 8

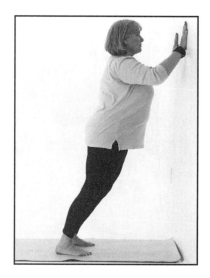

This is an optional step to be added after the second round. Bring the left foot back to meet the right as you lower the palms to the level of the shoulders. Bend the elbows, keep them tucked in toward the body, and press the pelvis toward the wall. Drop the shoulders away from the ears and try to feel a squeeze between the shoulder blades. This is an adapted version of the traditional cobra pose (page 78) and it is a little challenging. If it's not comfortable for you, feel free to omit it.

Position 9

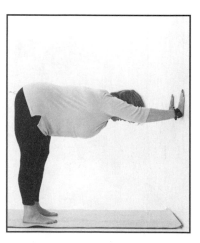

Come back into the wall dog by walking the hands down the wall until they reach hip level. Check to see that the arms are alongside the ears, to protect the neck. Keep the knees soft, with just a hint of a bend, or bend them a little more for comfort. Lengthen and soften the back of the neck.

Position 10

Push away from the wall and come into a standing forward bend. Keep the legs soft and hang the head and the arms.

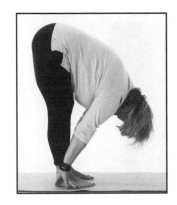

Position 11

a. Exhale as you bend the knees and begin to drop the buttocks down into a squat. Sweep the arms up so they come alongside the ears—if you find the wall is getting in the way, you may have to move back a little. Look down toward the floor, allowing the back of the neck to lengthen. Hold for a couple breaths.

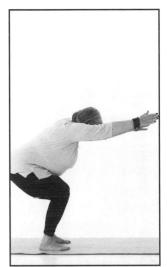

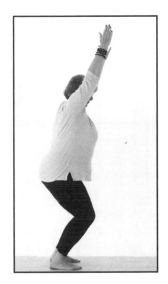

b. Inhale as you begin to straighten the knees. Keep the arms alongside the ears as you raise yourself up 75 percent of the way into the chair pose. Be careful to keep the knees in alignment with the feet and hips so they don't get knock-kneed, which is very hard on them.

c. Come all the way up to a standing position. The arms will naturally come up, too, if you keep them alongside the ears. Clasp the fingers overhead and relax the shoulders down.

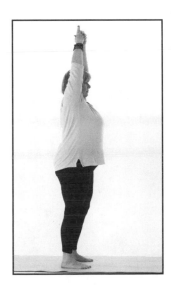

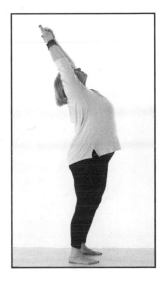

d. Gently bend backward on an exhale, feeling a little squeeze along the bottom of the shoulder blades. Inhale back up to standing position, and exhale as you begin to release the arms down.

Position 12

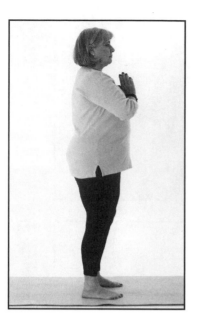

Inhale as you bring the palms together under the chin. Close the eyes, spread the feet, and let the arms drop alongside the body. Relax. When the breath returns to normal, continue for two more rounds.

Salute to the Sun
CHAIR ADAPTATION

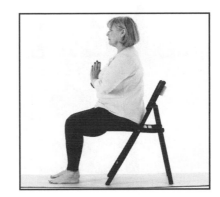

Position 1

Sit in a chair with the buttocks close to the front edge and the feet flat on the floor, about a foot apart. Place the palms together under the chin. Feel the spine getting longer and the shoulders getting wider.

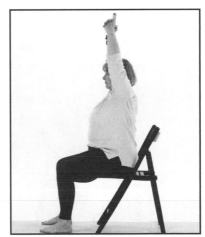

Position 2

Inhale and stretch the arms out to the sides, then up overhead. Keep the head between the arms and the shoulders relaxed and down. To enhance the stretch, exhale and arch the body back slightly, opening up the chest.

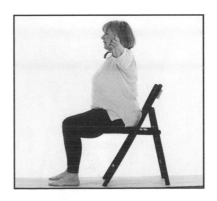

Position 3

Inhale and stretch up again. Then, exhale and begin to sweep the arms down to the sides and bend forward, engaging the abdominal muscles.

Position 4

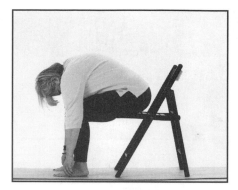

Relax forward, bringing the head down and softening the back of the neck. If this is too much of a strain, bring the hands up to the knees for support and ease up on the forward bend.

Position 5

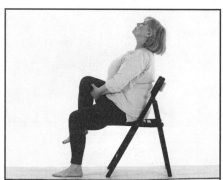

Inhale as you sit up. Draw the right knee up to the chest and take hold of the leg under the knee with the hands, giving yourself a hug. Have a slight lift in the chin, allowing the chest to expand, and draw the shoulders slightly back as you hold for a few breaths.

Position 6

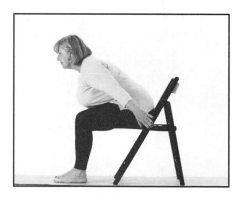

Inhale and release the right leg, bringing the right foot back down to the floor and sitting up tall. Sweep both arms behind the body on an exhalation and feel a squeeze at the bottom of the shoulder blades as you bend forward from the hips like a hinge.

Position 7

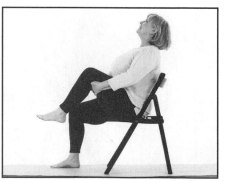

Inhale and begin to sit up as you re-peat the sequence with the left knee drawn up toward the chest. Keep a lift in the spine as you con-tinue to hug the knee into the chest for a few more breaths.

Inhale and release the left leg, bringing the left foot back down to the floor. Sweep both arms behind the body as you bend forward on an exhalation and feel a squeeze at the bottom of the shoulder blades.

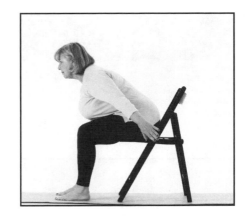

Position 8

Inhale as you sit up and bring the arms overhead, alongside the ears.

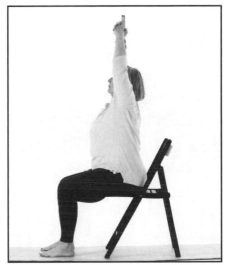

Position 9

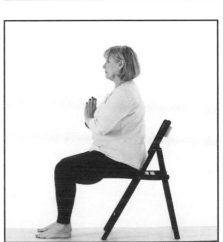

Position 10

Exhale and bring the arms down. Place the palms together at the heart center. Close the eyes and feel the effects of your practice. Repeat three or more times for an excellent warm up.

3. Supine Corpse
Savaasana

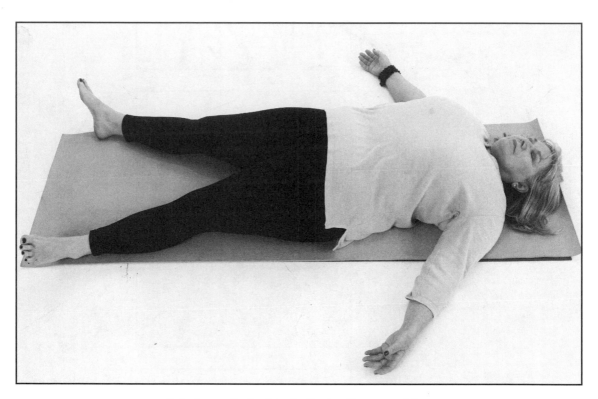

Relaxing on the back in the Supine Corpse position.

BENEFIT

Although you wouldn't really call the supine corpse pose a "warm-up," I have in-cluded it here because it is such an important part of the *Big Yoga* session. It is often done between poses or groups of poses to give the body a chance to assim-ilate the benefits, to "right" itself, and for deep relaxation—Yoga Nidra.

TECHNIQUE

Lie on your back with the feet at least a foot apart. Close the eyes and feel them softening in the sockets. Have the arms at a 45-degree angle from the torso, with the palms facing up. Roll the shoulders back and down slightly. Feel the floor sup-porting the weight of the body, and feel your body releasing and letting go. If you sense that you're holding on somewhere, tense that part of the body for a moment. Give it a good squeeze, and then quickly release it. Each time you come into the supine corpse during your Yoga session, you'll find that you're able to let go a little bit more and release into stillness.

DURATION

Beginner: During your Yoga session, the corpse position is recommended between each of the floor poses, for as long as it takes for the breath to come back to normal. During Yoga Nidra, which is often done at the end of an asana session, it can be held anywhere from five minutes to half an hour.

Intermediate: As you gain in expertise, you can shorten the time of resting between the floor poses, or skip the corpse until you feel the need to take a break. Listen to your own body and follow its cues.

ADAPTATION

Place a pillow under the head or the small of the back for more comfort. A bolster—a fat pillow in the shape of a tootsie-roll—also releases tension in the small of the back when placed under the knees.

4. Prone Corpse
Advaasana

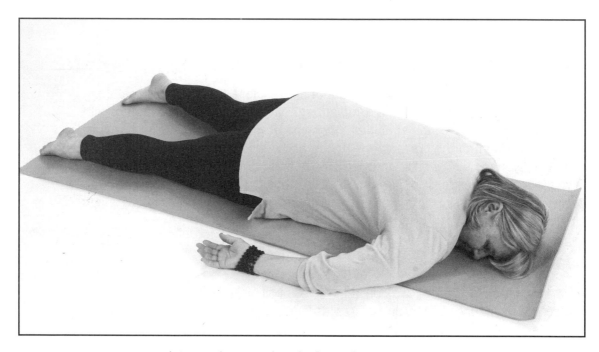

Lying on the stomach in the Prone Corpse position.

BENEFIT

The benefits of the prone corpse pose are the same as for the supine corpse pose (page 63).

TECHNIQUE

Lie on the belly with the legs wide and the arms resting alongside the body, palms up. Turn the head to one side and rest the cheek on the floor. As you inhale, feel the back ribs expanding, allowing the breath to fill the lungs. If you prefer, you can brings the arms overhead with elbows bent, as if you were taking a nap.

DURATION

Beginner: Use this as a resting pose between the prone floor poses in your Yoga session. When the breath returns to normal, go on to the next pose in the sequence.

Intermediate: If you've been practicing regularly, you may not need to rest in this pose very long, if at all.

CONSIDERATION

If you carry your weight in the belly or breasts, this may not be a restful position for you. If this is the case, instead try the reclining Buddha pose (page 66).

ADAPTATION

Put a small book under your cheek to raise the head slightly for comfort.

5. Reclining Buddha

Sayana Buddhasana

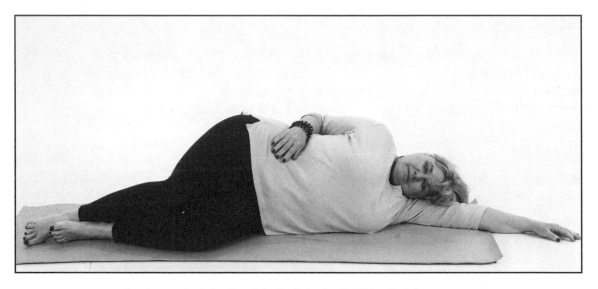

Resting on the left side of the body in the Reclining Buddha posture.

BENEFIT

The reclining Buddha makes a good resting pose when the corpse poses aren't comfortable for your body. In addition, lying on the left side of the body helps the breath to flow more readily in and out of the right nostril, which increases heat in the system and helps burn impurities.

TECHNIQUE

Lying on the floor, come onto the left side of the body and rest with the left arm overhead and the head on the left arm. Bring the right arm in front of the body with the palm on the floor for support. The left leg is extended in line with the body. The right leg is slightly bent and draped over the left, with the knee dropping down toward the floor. This pose is especially helpful if you carry a lot of weight in your belly and are uncomfortable in the prone corpse pose.

DURATION

Beginner: Generally, this pose is used as a brief transition between the floor asanas when lying prone is uncomfortable. It can also be used as a stand-alone asana anytime you need a rest but don't have time to go to sleep.

Intermediate: Experiment with the reclining Buddha and see if it fits into your practice. Use as needed.

6. Cat Pose

Biralasana

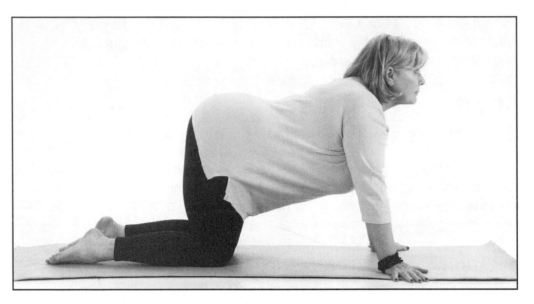

The first part of the Cat Pose, with the chin and
tailbone lifted, with the belly sinking toward the floor.

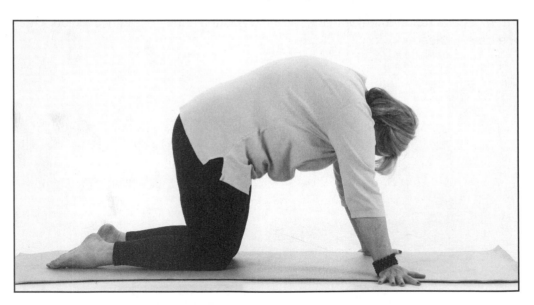

The second part of the Cat Pose, with the chin to the
chest, the spine rounded, and the tailbone tucked down.

BENEFIT

The cat pose helps to warm-up the spine and get you ready to move into the forward and backward bends.

TECHNIQUE

Come onto your mat on all fours, in the "table-top" position. The knees should be directly under the hips and the palms under the shoulders. Inhaling, draw the chin upward, lift the tailbone, and let the middle of the spine droop down. Exhale and bring the chin to chest, round the spine, and tuck the tailbone. The highest part of the arch should be the bottom of the shoulder blades. Try to keep the hips over the knees and not let them drift forward. At the end of the exhalation, draw the belly up to the spine. As soon as you feel the breath wanting to come back in, repeat the first position.

DURATION

Beginner: The movement should follow the breath—Inhale into position one and exhale into position two (sometimes called "the cow"). Don't hold the breath, rather, keep it fluid. Do three or four repetitions.

Intermediate: If you would like to gently hold the breath between each position, try that. As you hold the pose, look for places in the body that can release and open. Three to five repetitions are recommended.

ADAPTATION

If your wrists are delicate, consider trying one or more of these variations. I like to come onto the pads at the base of my fingers and use them for support, which solves the wrist problem. Another idea is to spread the hands a little wider than shoulder-width apart, point the fingers out so that they are perpendicular to the torso, and have a slight bend in the elbows. Or, make fists and come onto the knuckles.

7. Happy Baby

Prasanna Shishu

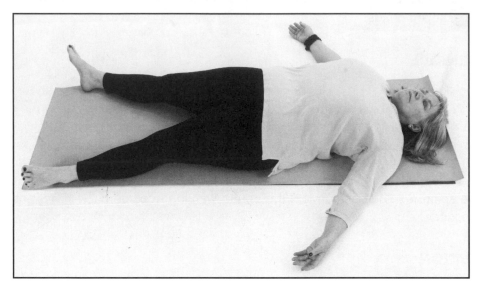

Begin on the back in the Supine Corpse.

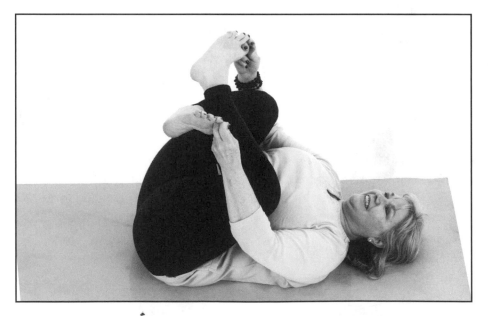

Enjoy the Happy Baby pose, and then return to the Supine Corpse.

BENEFIT

The happy baby warms up both the spine and the muscles surrounding and supporting the hip joint. When we carry extra weight, the hips can become fatigued. This pose takes all the pressure off of them, and the elevation of the legs helps to refresh the entire pelvic area.

TECHNIQUE

Begin on the floor in the supine corpse. Draw both knees up to the chest and rock from side to side to open up the lumbar spine. Cross the feet at the ankles and grab the opposite foot with each hand. Again rock from side to side, and then try to make circles with the hips, in both directions. Finally, rock top to bottom. After you get a little momentum, see if you can rock all the way up to a seated position. (Whee!) Alternatively, once you've got hold of the feet, relax the legs completely and just rest, feeling the muscles of the inner thighs "melting" and softening. To come out of the pose, release the legs back to the floor with control, either one at a time or simultaneously.

DURATION

Beginner: One long round, held for a few minutes at the end during the "melting," is recommended.

Intermediate: Same as for beginners.

CONSIDERATION

Be careful not to jerk your body into or out of this pose, so you don't throw anything out of alignment. Use the strength of your abdominal muscles to bring the legs up and down to the floor.

ADAPTATION

It's not necessary to take hold of the opposite foot. If it seems more comfortable to take hold of the right foot with the right hand, and the left foot with the left hand, try that.

8. Rock the Baby
Dolaayaate Shishu

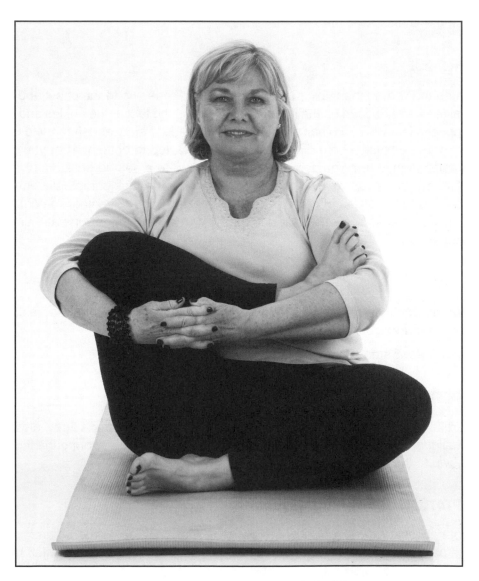

Hugging the leg into the chest in the Rock the Baby pose.

BENEFIT

This pose helps to open the hips, as well as massage the hips and buttocks. It also creates a feeling of self-nurturing as you hug the leg.

TECHNIQUE

Sit cross-legged on the floor and lift through the spine. Slide the right hand down the right leg and pick up the foot at the ankle. Draw the leg toward the left arm and place the foot into the crook of the left elbow, or somewhere near it. Cradle the leg with both arms and rock it gently from side to side, giving a stretch to the muscles that support the hip joint. To release, slide the hands down the right leg as you stretch it out in front of you. Slowly release the hands, and bring the leg back to the floor. Repeat on the other side. This constitutes one round.

DURATION

Beginner: One to three rounds, rocking each leg about three to five times, are fine.

Intermediate: Same as for beginners.

CONSIDERATION

Be sure to stay lifted through the spine during this pose, even if it means you can't bring the foot up very high.

ADAPTATION

If you're not comfortable on the floor, try sitting on a chair. Follow the rest of the directions as they are listed above.

Backward Bends

Now that we've warmed up the body a little with the salute to the sun and other warm-up exercises, we'll offer a variety of backward bends. The poses in this section are done on the belly, which gives a nice toning to the abdominal organs. In addition, they help lengthen the spine and tone the muscles supporting it. Be sure to follow the backbends with a stretch in the opposite direction during your own personal practice. As you will see, several forward bends are offered beginning on page 89 for this purpose.

9. Sphinx

12. Backward Boat
   Poorva Nauaasana

10. Cobra
   Bhujangaasana

13. Bow
   Dhanuraasana

11. Half Locust
   Arddha
   Salabaasana

14. Raised Bow
   Utthitha
   Dhanuraasana

9. Sphinx

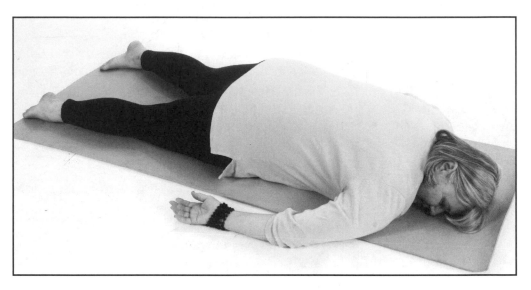

Begin in the Prone Corpse position.

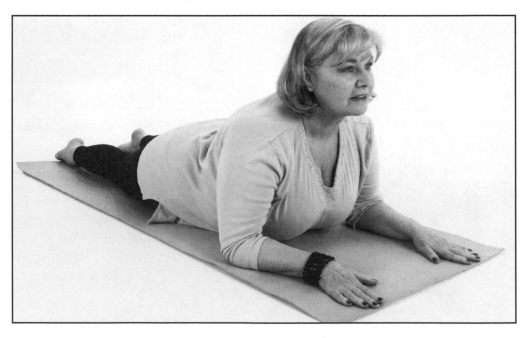

Raise up into the Sphinx pose, and then lower back down into the Prone Corpse.

BENEFIT

A good preparation for the cobra (page 78), the sphinx stretches the chest, lungs, and spine. It also stimulates the abdominal organs and has a calming effect on the entire system.

TECHNIQUE

Lying on the floor in the prone corpse, bring the feet together with the toes pointing away from the body, and feel the tops of the feet pressing softly into the floor. Imagine the tailbone lengthening toward the feet, and the sacrum—the hard, bony, triangular structure at the back of the pelvis—broadening, as well. Place the upper-arms alongside the body with the elbows in line with the shoulders. Bring the forearms forward and parallel to each other, with the palms face down. Inhale and lift your head and chest as you come into a gentle backbend. Gaze forward and soften the back of the neck. Relax the legs and feel the lower back sinking toward the floor. Exhale as you come out of the pose by gracefully lowering the chest and head to the floor. Turn the cheek to the one side and rest in the prone corpse, feeling the muscles supporting the vertebrae softening and relaxing with each exhalation.

DURATION

Beginner: Hold for up to five breaths and exhale down. If you like, you can do one or two more repetitions.

Intermediate: Hold for five to ten breaths and exhale down. When you're able to hold the pose longer, you don't need to do any repetitions—unless you're really enjoying it!

CONSIDERATION

Be careful not to let the shoulders shrug up toward the ears during this exercise. If you carry your weight in your belly and it feels like it's getting scrunched up in the area between the navel and the pubic bone, lift the torso, and shift the ribs forward. Or, you might try lifting and lowering the legs, one at a time, to smooth out the belly. Refrain from doing this pose if you are bothered by a headache or recent back injury.

10. Cobra
Bhujangaasana

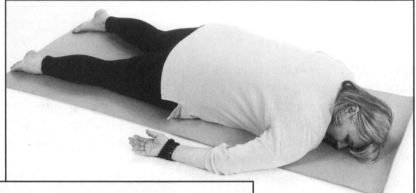

Begin on the stomach in the Prone Corpse.

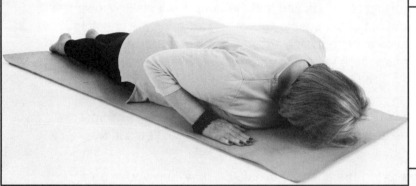

Bring the feet together, the forehead to the floor, and the palms under the shoulders.

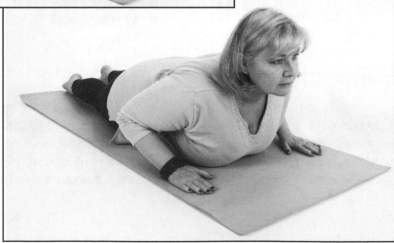

Raise the head, neck, and chest off the floor into the Cobra pose.

BENEFIT

The cobra pose opens the chest, exercises the upper back muscles, and gives a fresh supply of blood to the cranial nerves. It is especially helpful for backache caused by sitting at a desk too long. This pose also gives a nice massage to the belly, toning the viscera and relieving gas and constipation.

TECHNIQUE

Lie on the floor in the prone corpse. Bring the feet together or slightly apart, and rest the forehead on the floor. Place the palms on the floor directly under the shoulders (near the armpits), with the elbows slightly raised and tucked in toward the torso. Keeping the legs relaxed, begin to slowly raise the head, neck, and chest, using the strength of the upper back rather than pushing up with the palms. Initiate the movement with an inhale, and then continue breathing throughout. Concentrate on trying to feel a backward curve at the bottom of the shoulder blades. To release, lower the body down slowly as you exhale, bringing the chin, nose, and forehead to the floor before resting in the supine corpse, with the cheek to the side.

DURATION

Beginner: Hold for up to three breaths, and then come out of the pose, leaving the hands in place while relaxing the legs and arms and turning the cheek to the side. Rest briefly. Then, come back to the preparatory stage, with the forehead on the floor and the arms and legs in place. Inhale as you come up for a second round, hold, and exhale down.

Intermediate: If you're able to hold the pose longer than three breaths, you only need to do one round. Simply hold for up to eight breaths without strain, and exhale down.

CONSIDERATION

Resist the temptation to push with the hands to get into position. Bring the hands up off the floor to check and see if you are truly using the strength of the upper back. Also, be sure to keep the legs soft throughout the entire exercise.

11. Half Locust
Arddha Salabaasana

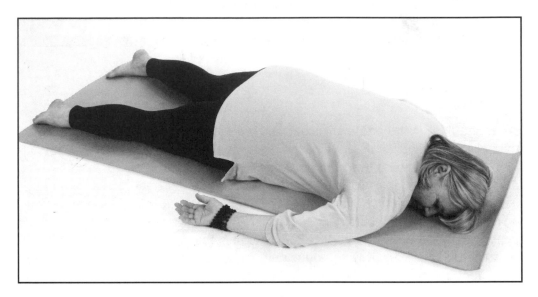

Begin in the Prone Corpse position.

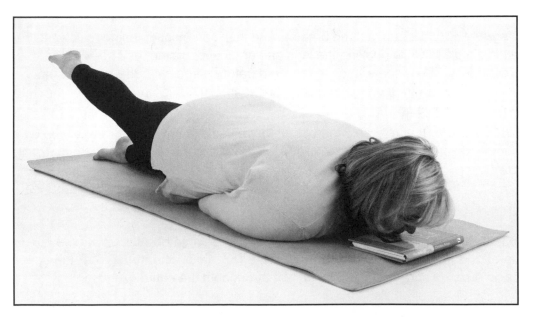

Bring the arms under the body, the chin to the floor,
and then extend and raise one leg at a time off the floor.

BENEFIT

The half locust tones the female organs by bringing a fresh supply of blood to the pelvic area. It also exercises the lower back muscles and gently massages the belly. Additionally, this pose tones the sympathetic nervous system and stimulates the liver into performing its functions more effectively.

TECHNIQUE

Starting in the prone corpse, place the chin directly on the floor. Bring the legs closer together, straighten the arms down by the sides, and slide them under the body. Lock the thumbs together under the thighs, with the palms up. Try to get the elbows as close together as possible by rocking gently from side to side. Then, begin to stretch out the right leg. Point the right foot at the ankle, extending the point through the toes. Inhale and raise the leg up off the floor, imagining someone is pulling on the big toe. Exhale slowly and lower the leg. Relax, and then repeat with the other leg.

DURATION

Beginner: Hold for a few breaths, no longer than is comfortable. If you can, do two repetitions on each side.

Intermediate: Begin to hold the pose longer, for up to five breaths. Once you are able to do two long repetitions, you can try doing the full locust, in which both legs come up off the floor at the same time.

CONSIDERATION

Be aware of alignment, and keep the hips parallel to the floor. Furthermore, be careful not to raise the legs too high. It's more important to have the raised leg steady and long than it is to have it high. And rest assured, you will still get the benefit even if you only raise the leg an inch or two off the ground.

ADAPTATION

If you carry your weight in the upper chest, you may find the chin is "floating" when lying on the belly. If this is the case, place a small hardcover book or block under the chin for support.

12. Backward Boat

Poorva Nauaasana

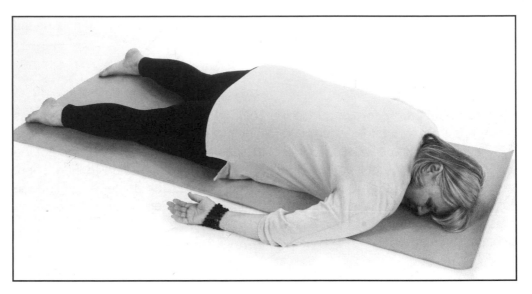

Begin in the Prone Corpse position.

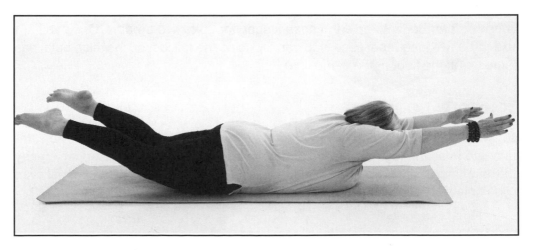

Raise up into the Backward Boat, with the weight resting on the belly.

BENEFIT

The backward boat is good for making the trunk of the body strong and solid. It is a good preparatory pose for the bow (page 84).

TECHNIQUE

Lie on the belly in the prone corpse. Bring the feet together and the arms over-head—palms facing down like a flying superman. Inhale and raise both halves of the body so that all the weight is resting on the belly. Hold without straining until you need to exhale, and then slowly do so while lowering everything down.

DURATION

Beginner: Repeat three to five times, inhaling up and exhaling down with each round.

Intermediate: As you gain strength, inhale up into the pose, and then continue to breathe normally as you hold the pose for three to five breaths. Exhale down, inhale up again, and repeat for up to five rounds.

CONSIDERATION

Remember that all movements in Yoga are done slowly and deliberately. Don't jerk the body up or down. In addition, don't hold the breath.

13. Bow

Dhanuraasana

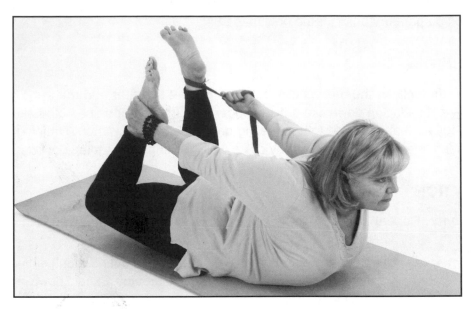

The Traditional Bow pose, using a strap as an extension on one leg.

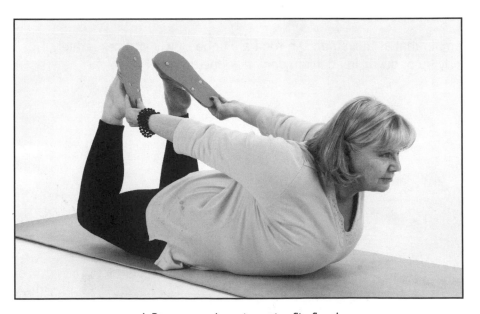

A Bow pose adaptation using flip-flops!

BENEFIT

The bow pose keeps the spine flexible and combines the benefit of the cobra and half locust poses (pages 78 and 80 respectively). Additionally, it tones the pancreas so it is helpful if you have diabetes, and it massages the belly, thereby reducing belly fat and keeping the bowels moving.

TECHNIQUE

Resting comfortably on the belly, bend the knees and reach back with both hands to take hold of the feet or the ankles. (Right hand grabbing right foot; left hand grabbing left foot.) Bring the forehead to the floor in a preparatory position. Activate the tops of the thighs, pressing them into the floor. Inhale and begin to raise the head, chest, and thighs off the floor to the best of your ability, without forcing the lift. Keep the arms straight, and allow the body to rock gently back and forth with the inhalations and exhalations. To come out of the pose, exhale and lower the thighs and chest to the floor with control. Bring the forehead back to the floor, draw circles in the air with the feet in both directions to rotate the ankles, and then gently release the legs with control. Rest in the prone corpse (page 64).

DURATION

Beginner: Hold for about ten seconds initially, and do one or two repetitions. Between repetitions, bring the forehead to the floor and relax the legs, but don't release the grip on the ankles or feet.

Intermediate: Stay in this pose anywhere from ten to thirty seconds. Relax the head and thighs to the floor as you exhale, and lie quietly for a few breaths. You can repeat the pose once or twice more.

CONSIDERATION

This pose is not recommended for those with uncontrolled high blood pressure, hernia, or ulcer of the stomach or intestine.

ADAPTATION

If you find you can't quite reach your ankles, you can use a strap or a tie to "lasso" your feet. Another trick I have used is to wear a pair of flip-flops and grab onto the heel of the shoes, which provides a little extension.

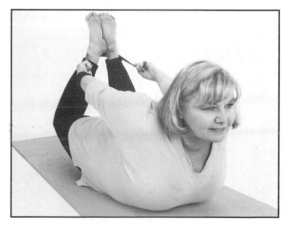

A Bow pose adaptation using a strap to "lasso" both legs.

14. Raised Bow

Utthitha Dhanuraasana

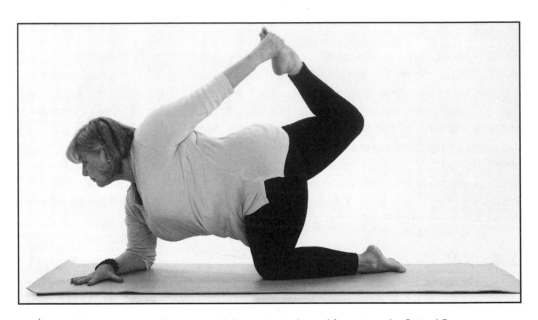

Balancing on one forearm and the opposite knee, life up into the Raised Bow.

BENEFIT

The raised bow improves balance and increases the spine's flexibility. It is often suggested for pregnant women, as it places no pressure on the abdomen.

TECHNIQUE

Begin on all fours with your knees directly below your hips and your hands directly below your shoulders, in a "table-top" position. Bring the right forearm down to the floor—perpendicular to the body—and put your weight on it. Bring the right foot toward the left, then up over the left calf, so you can see the right foot behind you when looking over the left shoulder. Take hold of the right foot with the left hand. Inhale as you gradually, bring the right foot up and back into alignment with the right shoulder and hip. Balance the weight on the right forearm and the left knee. When you feel steady, try arching the back and lifting the head, chest, and right foot. Exhale as you release in the same order, allowing the right foot to come back over to the left calf before you release. Repeat on the other side.

DURATION

Beginner: Generally, this pose is only done once on each side.

Intermediate: Repeat if you like.

CONSIDERATION

Be careful not to let your bow "snap!" When releasing the feet, the movements should be controlled and steady.

ADAPTATION

If your knees are sensitive, support them by placing a folded blanket or an extra layer of mat underneath them.

Forward Bends

When you practice Yoga's physical postures, it's important to balance the body by stretching it in all different directions: backward and forward, side to side, and even upside down! This section on forward bends is the compliment to the last section on backward bends. However, in your personal practice, it's not necessary to do every pose in these two sections. You might want to choose one or two backbends, and then follow with one or two forward bends. Then, the next time you do Yoga, select a different backbend and an alternate forward bend. The more you mix it up, the better results you'll have. Think of the forward bends as surrendering poses. Enjoy the feeling of release, rather than forcing yourself to achieve a certain position.

15. Head-to-Knee Pose
   Janusirshaasana

18. Child's Pose
   Balasaana

16. Full Forward Bend
   Paschimothanaasana

19. Yogic Seal
   Yoga Mudra

17. Standing Forward
   Bend
   Uttasaana

15. Head-to-Knee Pose
Janusirshaasana

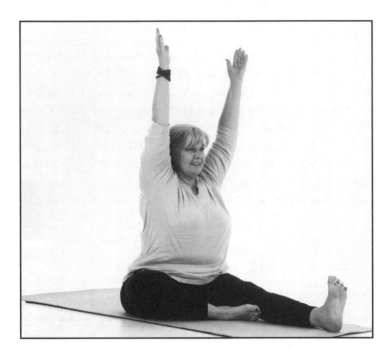

Begin by stretching the arms and torso upwards, lengthening the spine.

Bend forward from the hips and relax into the Head-To-Knee pose.

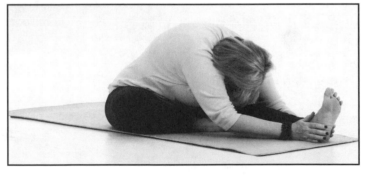

BENEFIT

The head-to-knee pose gives a good stretch to the posterior muscles. It also gives a nice massage to the belly and its internal organs. When we squeeze the organs in this way, we force out toxins, like wringing out water from a sponge. Upon release, fresh blood will immediately flow back into the organs, refreshing them and bringing more vitality into the subtle systems of the body.

TECHNIQUE

Sit on the floor with both legs outstretched in front of you. Bend the left leg and place the left heel against the inside of the right leg. Check to see that the right foot is aligned with the right leg, which in turn is aligned with the right hip and right shoulder. Flex the right foot with the toes pointing up. Inhale and stretch the arms and torso upwards, lengthening the spine. Exhale and bend forward from the hips like a hinge. Place the hands at a comfortable place along the outstretched leg, or rest them comfortably on the knee. Allow the head to drop forward, bringing the forehead closer to the knee. Relax into the pose. Try to keep the right foot flexed, being careful not to let it flop to one side. To come out of the pose, stretch just a little further, inhale, and come up, keeping the arms alongside the ears, locking the thumbs if you like. Then, bring the hands to the lap and repeat on the other side. When you've done both sides, release the arms and stretch both legs out in front of you. Once again, stretch the arms overhead, lock the thumbs, and exhale as you lower the body back to the floor vertebra by vertebra to rest in the supine corpse (page 62).

DURATION

Beginner: One repetition is all that is needed. Hold the pose only as long as you are comfortable, for no longer than five breaths. After you have held the pose for a few breaths, you may find you can stretch a little further forward. Make the adjustment, but then become still and enjoy the stretch.

Intermediate: Feel free to hold the pose up to eight long breaths. Once on each side is all you need.

CONSIDERATION

Keep the arms and shoulders relaxed. A larger belly can create an obstacle to bending deeply into the pose, so try placing the hands at the knees in the beginning. If you find the breathing becomes labored because of belly fat, back off the pose a little until you find your comfort zone. Remember, you'll still get the benefits of the pose even when you don't look like the picture.

ADAPTATION

Placing a pillow or folded blanket under the buttocks to slightly elevate the hips will make you more comfortable. You can also soften the knee of the outstretched leg to create a slight bend if that's more comfortable, but be sure to maintain correct alignment.

16. Full Forward Bend

Paschimothanaasana

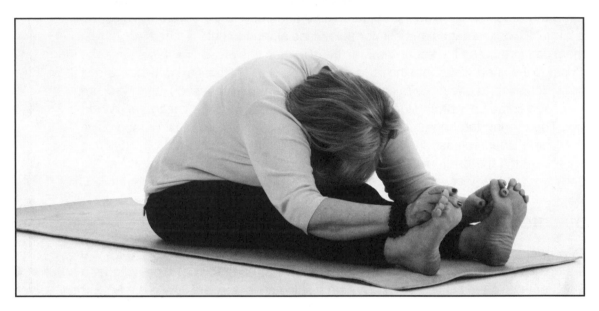

Release into the Full Forward Bend.

BENEFIT

The full forward bend exercises the posterior muscles and tones up the abdominal viscera, or what we may call the "guts." It's a good antidote to sitting in a chair all day, which tends to cause these muscles to atrophy. It also helps reduce abdominal fat and prevent menstrual disorders by gently squeezing and toning the belly and female organs in that area. Furthermore, this pose is beneficial in lowering blood pressure and cortisol, the stress hormone.

TECHNIQUE

In a seated position with both legs outstretched in front of you, "rearrange" the buttocks so that the sit bones are freely connected to the floor. Inhale and stretch the arms overhead, locking thumbs if you like. Keeping the arms alongside the ears, exhale down, bending forward from the hips—like a hinge—for a full forward release. Place the hands at a comfortable place on the legs. For beginners, placing them on your knees is fine. In time and with practice, you will gain flexibility and be able to bring the hands down closer to the ankles, then to the feet, and ultimately, to the toes. When your hands are situated, fully release into the pose. Think about the breath as you continue holding it. Inhale fresh energy into the body, and send it to any place that is giving resistance. Then, slowly exhale all negativity out of the body, through the breath. To come out of the pose, stretch the arms forward, lock thumbs if you like, inhale, and come up, keeping the arms beside the ears. Keep the entire spine lifted throughout, and the legs soft. When you come back to a seated position, use the abdominal muscles to roll backwards into the supine corpse (page 62).

DURATION

Beginner: Try holding for three to five breaths if that's comfortable. One repetition is fine.

Intermediate: Holding the pose for three to eight breaths is fine, as long as there is no strain. When we hold the poses longer, there's no need for a second round unless you are working on a specific problem, such as gaining flexibility in the backs of the legs.

CONSIDERATION

Although short retention of this pose helps to prevent constipation, if you are constipated, don't hold this pose too long. Additionally, this pose is not recommended for people with abdominal problems. The forward bends are considered surrendering poses, so make sure you relax the effort until you are really comfortable. Having a slight bend in the knees can often make the forward bends more comfortable.

ADAPTATION

If you carry your weight in the belly and the traditional forward bend is uncomfortable, try placing a large bolster between your legs and, bending from the hips, folding forward over the bolster. Allow the hands to find a comfortable place on top of the bolster and relax the arms. This can also be done without the bolster, with the legs spread wide.

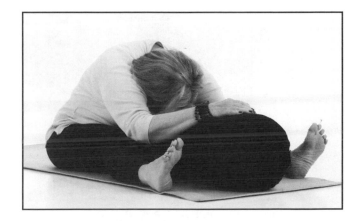

Full Forward Bend adaptation using a bolster.

17. Standing Forward Bend
Uttaasana

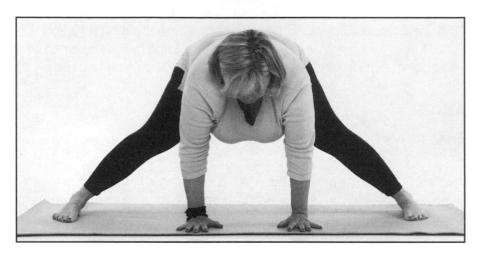

Coming into the Standing Forward Bend, releasing the hands down toward the floor.

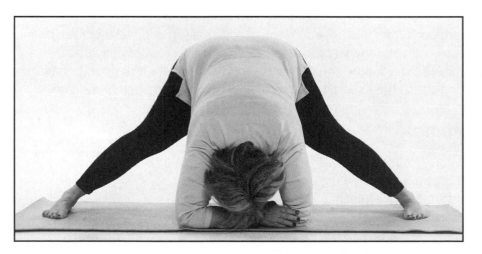

Relaxing the neck, head, and arms in the Standing Forward Bend.

BENEFIT

The standing forward bend stretches the hamstrings (the back of the thighs) and aligns the hips and legs. It also invigorates your whole system by inverting the upper body, which allows bodily fluids to reverse their flow.

TECHNIQUE

Stand with the feet about three feet apart from one another and place the hands on the hips. Exhale and bend forward, hinging at the hips. As the head gets closer to the floor, release the hands down toward it. Relax the neck and let the head and arms hang loosely. To come out of this pose, bring the feet about a foot apart and bend the knees slightly so the belly is resting on the thighs. Cross the arms in front of the body so the head is between them. Slowly, with control, curl the body up to a standing position, having slow, deliberate breaths. At a certain point, which varies from individual to individual, your arms will automatically release. Allow that to happen naturally and continue to come up, keeping the chin tucked gently into the chest until you're all the way up. Take a moment to rest in the mountain pose (page 123).

DURATION

Beginner: Once you are in the pose, hold for a few breaths and come out of it slowly. One round is enough for a beginner.

Intermediate: If you're really flexible, try bringing the forearms to the floor, perpendicular to the body, and separate the feet a little wider. Come up as directed. One round is enough even for the intermediate student, but hold the pose a little longer—up to eight breaths—before coming up.

CONSIDERATION

This pose is not recommended if you are suffering from a headache.

ADAPTATION

Depending on flexibility, this pose can be adapted by using blocks, a table, or a chair as support for the extended arms.

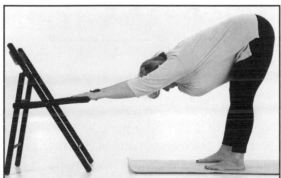

Adaptation using a chair as support.

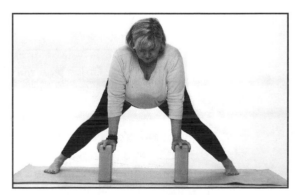

Adaptation using blocks as support.

18. Child's Pose

Balaasana

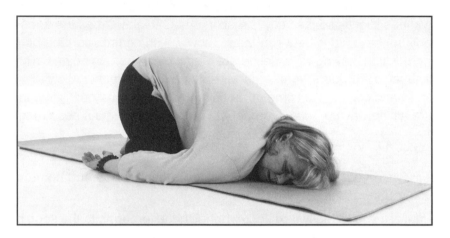

Child's pose with the arms alongside the body, palms up.

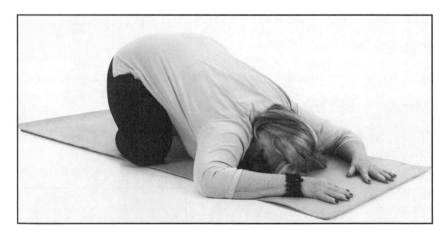

Child's pose with the arms overhead, palms down.

BENEFIT

The elevation of the hips during the child's pose draws energy down to the head and heart, giving them both a little rest. This pose also relieves the pain of menstrual cramps and can reduce excess energy and fluid during women's periods. It can also enhance circulation to the kidneys, adrenal glands, and spleen when the breath is directed to the lower back, which will occur over time, with practice.

TECHNIQUE

Begin on all fours with your knees directly below your hips and your hands directly below your shoulders, in the "table-top" position. Drop the buttocks back toward the feet and bring the forearms to the floor, perpendicular to the body, for support. Widen the stance of the knees to wherever you feel comfortable. Slide the arms down alongside the body, palms up, and turn the head to one side so the cheek is resting on the floor. Alternately, try stretching the arms forward over the head, palms down, reaching toward the top edge of the mat.

DURATION

Beginner: Child's pose is often done frequently throughout the Yoga session because of its relaxing effect. Add it into your practice whenever you feel the need to take a little break and stretch out the back. Hold for three to five breaths.

Intermediate: Hold for three to five breaths if you're using it as a resting pose between other exercises. Or, at the end of the Yoga session, it can be held for up to ten breaths in place of the Yogic seal (page 98).

CONSIDERATION

For those of us who carry extra weight, we need to take care not to strain in this pose. Remember, it is designed to be soothing. Keep experimenting with your own placement of arms, knees, and head until you feel yourself go "Aaaahhhhh."

ADAPTATION

If your knees are sensitive, support them by placing a folded blanket or an extra layer of mat underneath them. Additionally, if you find you need more support, you can place a large bolster, lengthwise, between the knees. Then, fold the body over it and hug the bolster. This adaptation is one of my favorite poses.

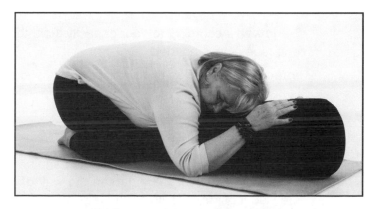

Child's pose adaptation using a bolster.

19. Yogic Seal
Yoga Mudra

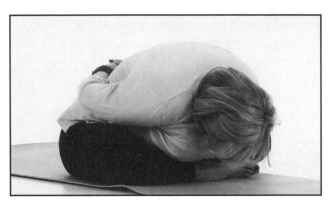

Bent forward in the Yogic Seal.

BENEFIT

The Yogic seal is traditionally done at the end of the asana practice because it seals the energy you've built up into the higher energy centers, or *chakras.* It also lowers the blood pressure and creates a wonderful sensation of reverence and peace.

TECHNIQUE

Sitting in a cross-legged position with the arms down by the sides, inhale as you bring the hands behind the lower back, taking hold of the left wrist with the right hand. Exhale, close the eyes, and bend forward from the hips, like a hinge. As soon as you've reached the edge of your comfort zone, release the head toward the earth and relax into the pose. To come out of it, slowly raise the trunk of the body on an inhale, leading with the chin. Keep the eyes closed and the awareness within. When your torso is erect, bring the hands to the knees and feel the effect of this powerful *mudra.*

DURATION

Beginner: According to your capacity, hold the pose for two to five breaths. Only one repetition is needed.

Intermediate: You can hold this pose for up to six breaths, but one round is all that is necessary.

ADAPTATION

If you can't grasp your wrist with your hand behind your back, use a strap or tie as an extender. If your belly gets in the way of a comfortable forward stretch with crossed legs, try stretching the legs out in front of you—spread wide—and come into the pose that way.

Inversions

When we turn the body upside down, all kinds of wonderful things begin to happen. The brain gets a fresh supply of blood that easily flows down from the heart. Also, the spent, or venous, blood that tends to pool at the feet drains effortlessly back to the heart for recirculation. The lymph system is also drained, allowing the body to fight off infection and disease. And the simple act of having the bones of the spine in an inverted position helps enhance alignment.

A special note to those diagnosed with diabetes: Some of the inversions can cause pressure to the eyes. If you have diabetes and/or have had retinal detachment, avoid poses that cause this pressure to build up. Check with your ophthalmologist to see if you are at risk and follow his or her advice.

20. Downward Dog
    Adho Mukha
    Svanaasana

21. Upright Legs
    Urdhva Prasarita
    Padaasana

22. Legs up the Wall/
    Shoulder Stand
    Viparita Karani/
    Sarvangaasana

23. Plow
    Halaasana

24. Fish
    Matsyaasana

25. Bridge
    Sethu Bandha
    Sarvangaasana

20. Downward Dog

Adho Mukha Svanaasana

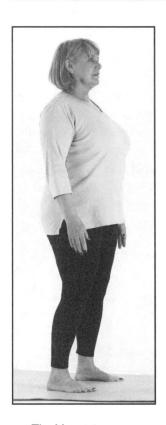

The Mountain pose.

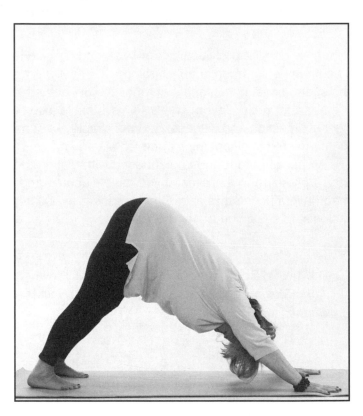

Performing the Downward Dog position.

BENEFIT

The downward dog provides an incredible stretch from the feet all the way up to the hips, as well as from the shoulders down through the wrists and hands. It lengthens the back of the legs including the ankles, calves, and hamstrings, and it activates the front of the thighs. Additionally, it engages the abdominal muscles, expands the chest, and stretches the lower back, shoulder blades, and arms. Even the joints of the fingers—especially where they join the palms—are activated by this pose. Furthermore, it increases circulation, especially to the brain. In short, the downward dog pose is rejuvenating and it strengthens the whole body.

TECHNIQUE

Standing in the mountain pose, begin to bend forward from the hips as you exhale. Bend the knees and bring the hands to the floor beside the feet. Step the right foot back and then the left, forming an inverted "V," with the tailbone as the apex. Stretch the heels toward the floor. Keep the head between the arms, or drop it a little lower if you can. Usually downward dog is done as a transitional pose, or even a resting pose, between other poses in a continuous flow, known as a *vinyasa*. If you're practicing it as a stand-alone pose, however, here's how to come out of it: Bend the knees slightly, and then walk the feet toward the hands and the hands toward the feet. When they come closer together, exhale, bend the knees, and drop the buttocks into a squat. Bring the arms alongside the ears, parallel to the floor with the palms facing each other. Hold for a moment, as you engage the thigh muscles. Begin to raise the torso up on an inhale, and come back into the mountain pose.

DURATION

Beginner: Downward dog is a classic pose that can be repeated several times during your Yoga session. When you are first beginning, hold it for up to five breaths.

Intermediate: Hold for up to eight deep breaths each time you come into this pose.

CONSIDERATION

Take care that the feet are parallel. Traditionally, the feet are together, but for the larger body, having the feet about six to twelve inches apart is preferable. If you have trouble with carpal tunnel syndrome, try coming up onto the pads at the base of the fingers. Or, try holding a block in each hand.

ADAPTATION

The wall adaptation of downward dog can be seen in the salute to the sun sequence (page 55). The "wall dog" is helpful for times when you want to have a nice stretch but can't—or don't want to—get down on the floor, such as during a bathroom break or a long trip on a plane. Another way to come into downward dog is to begin in a table-top position on your knees and hands. Simply curl the toes under and push up, raising the buttocks high on an inhale. Come out in reverse, on an exhale.

21. Upright Legs
Urdhva Prasarita Padaasana

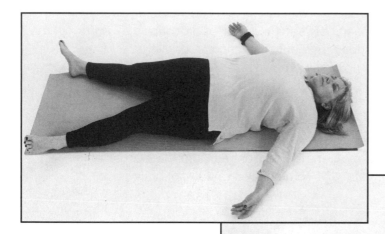

Begin in the Supine Corpse.

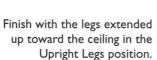

Finish with the legs extended up toward the ceiling in the Upright Legs position.

BENEFIT

This pose helps to tone the abdominal and back muscles, and is good preparation for other inverted poses.

TECHNIQUE

Starting in the supine corpse, turn the palms down and bring the hands close to the sides of the body. Bring the feet together and on an exhale, and then draw the knees up to the chest. Inhale and raise the legs up, extending them completely while keeping them aligned with the hips. Flex the feet, with the soles facing the ceiling. Continue with intentional breaths, and at the end of the exhalations, draw the belly toward the spine. If comfortable, bring the arms overhead to rest on the floor, palms up. Draw the shoulders down and away from the neck. Rest here for a few deep breaths, or more if you're able. To come out of the pose, bring the palms back to the floor next to the body for support, and slowly lower the legs back to the floor. If it's a little challenging to lower both legs simultaneously, do one at a time, with control. Work those abs!

DURATION

Beginner: To gain strength, hold for a few breaths and repeat for up to three rounds.

Intermediate: As you become stronger and are able to hold the pose for three to five long breaths, you only need to do one or two rounds.

CONSIDERATION

If you have mild sciatica, keep the knees bent. Or, for more acute sciatica, avoid this pose. If your lower back arches throughout the pose, don't hold it for very long. And if you find it's too challenging to bring both legs up and down simultaneously, raise and lower them one at a time.

ADAPTATION

If the upright legs pose seems a little challenging for you, place a chair at the foot of your mat. Beginning in the supine corpse, bend the knees and bring the feet close to the buttocks. Place the palms face-down a few inches away from the hips for support. Inhale and bring one leg up to rest the calf on the seat of the chair. When you feel steady, inhale and bring the other leg up in the same manner. Next, raise and straighten one leg so that it's perpendicular to the floor. You might want to hold there and do one leg at a time. Or, with practice, you can bring them both up. After a few breaths, lower the legs back to the chair in reverse order. Take a moment to rest with the calves on the seat of the chair, and then proceed to lower the legs back to the floor, one at a time.

22. Legs up the Wall/ Shoulder Stand

Viparita Karani/Sarvangaasana

BENEFIT

Most of us big folks can't do a traditional shoulder stand without throwing our legs up overhead and jerking our bodies in ways that can be harmful. Therefore, I have combined it with the legs up the wall pose, which is a good way to come into the shoulder stand without hurting yourself. It is also a stand-alone pose that is wonderfully restorative. Known as the "all members pose" for its beneficial effects on the whole body, the shoulder stand helps in curing asthma, all sorts of digestive problems, hernias, diabetes, and heart troubles. The thyroid gets a gentle massage in this pose, as well, stimulating the production of thyroxin and balancing the metabolism. It also has the effect of draining the lymph system, which is your body's "sewer." Unlike the circulatory system, the lymph system doesn't have a pump, so this pose helps to keep the lymph from stagnating. Try practicing the legs up the wall for several weeks before attempting the full shoulder stand, or even better, wait until you have a teacher to guide you into this more challenging, but worthwhile pose.

"Know the value of time. Time is most precious.
Utilize every second profitably.
Live every moment of your life for the
Realization of your ideal and goal.
Do not procrastinate. That "tomorrow" will never come.
Now or never. Abandon idle gossiping.
Kill egoism, laziness and inertia. Forget the past.
A glorious and brilliant future is awaiting you.
Be in tune with the Infinite."
MASTER SIVANANDA

TECHNIQUE

Stage 1

a. Sit beside a wall free of pictures and furniture, with the left hip against the wall and the legs extended out in front of you.

b. Place the right hand behind you for support, and begin to fall backward while you bring your legs up the wall. Swivel your body so that it is perpendicular to the wall and scoot your buttocks right up next to it. Take a moment to let the legs rest comfortably on the wall. Make sure you allow the breath to come back to normal before you continue.

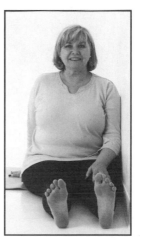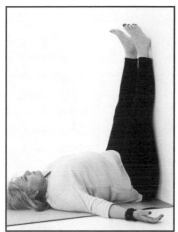

Stage 2

If you feel you can do more, bend the knees and place the feet flat against the wall. Push gently against the wall with the feet to lift the buttocks up off the floor. If you have long hair, pull it to either side so it doesn't get caught under the back of the neck. Try a few repetitions of this, and then rest with the legs or feet against the wall. If you feel comfortable with this stage, you can go on to the next.

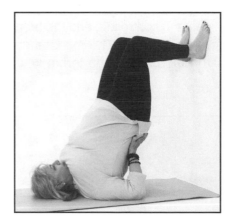

Stage 3

Again, press the feet against the wall and raise the buttocks off the floor. This time, though, bring the palms to the small of the back for support and bring the elbows a little closer together. The chin and the chest will naturally come closer together.

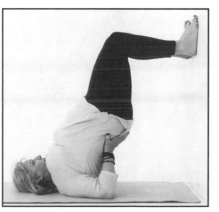

Stage 4

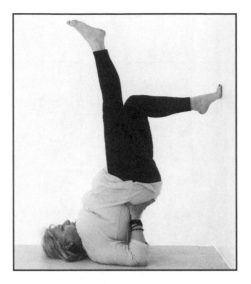 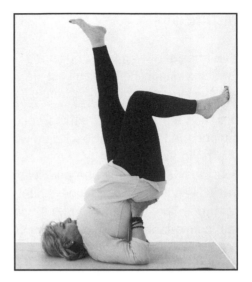

From the stage-three position, try bringing one leg off the wall at a time, taking care to keep the body balanced and controlled, and the breath gentle and deep. The focus should be on the base of the throat where the thyroid is located. Those of us with large breasts can avoid feeling smothered in this position by using a strap to bind the breasts, which helps keep them from falling onto the nose and mouth.

Stage 5

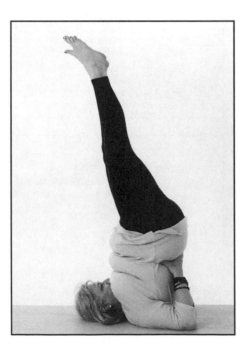

This stage is the full shoulder stand and it's not recommended without the guidance of a teacher. However, I'm showing it here so you have an idea of what you might want to work toward, since the benefits of the shoulder stand are considerable. Beginning in the stage-three pose, bring both legs off the wall with complete control. Once in position, relax, but continue to lengthen the legs and try to create a little more space between the ears and the tops of the shoulders. Bringing the elbows closer together helps to give you a good solid stance.

Recovery

To come out of this pose, go in the reverse order. First bring one foot back to the wall, then the other. Release the hands from the lower back and slowly begin to lower the body down, vertebra by vertebra, bringing the arms alongside the body with the palms down for support. Once the buttocks are back on the floor and the legs are straightened against the wall, swing the legs back down. Pause for fifteen to twenty seconds to allow the breath to return to normal, and then allow the torso to pop back up. Or, alternately, roll to the side in a fetal position, rest awhile, and come up at your own pace.

DURATION

Beginner: Practice stage one for a few sessions before going on to stage two, and so on. One round, held for up to three breaths at each stage, is all that is recommended.

Intermediate: Please take care not to overdo it, but when you feel you have the strength to hold the different stages for up to six breaths, do that. Again, I would emphasize that you should consult a Yoga teacher before doing the full shoulder stand.

CONSIDERATION

Don't "throw" your legs from the wall, which may throw you off balance. Try not to sneeze, swallow, or cough while the legs are up overhead. Keep the breath slow and steady, with no retention. When coming out of this pose, take your time so as not to get lightheaded. Do not practice this pose if you have a headache, and please check with your doctor if you have high blood pressure.

23. Plow

Halaasana

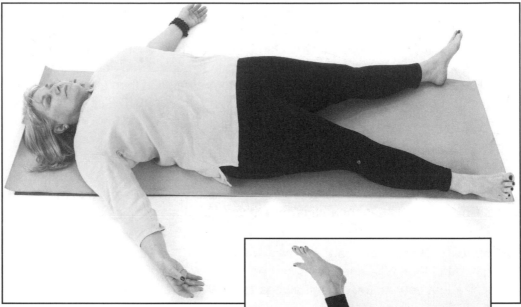

One option is to begin in the Supine Corpse.

BENEFIT

This pose is beneficial for gaining flexibility in the spine and bringing nourishment to the nerves along the spine. Additionally, like the shoulder stand, it tones the thyroid gland. Practiced regularly, the plow pose can help reduce abdominal fat and improve diabetic conditions, constipation, indigestion, and rheumatism.

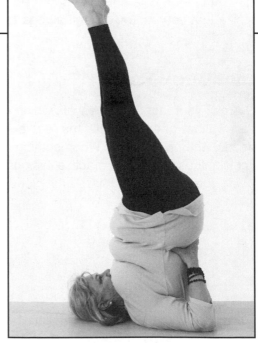

Another option is to begin in the Shoulder Stand.

TECHNIQUE

When coming out of the shoulder stand, after some practice, try coming into the plow. Before bringing the legs back to the wall, lower the hands down to the floor for support, and exhale as you allow the legs to lower down over the head toward the floor. Keep the weight of the body on the shoulders, not the neck. All movement should be controlled and fluid, not jerky. Rather than holding this pose, do a few repetitions—especially if you are still new to practicing Yoga. This pose can also be performed separate from the shoulder stand, coming out of the supine corpse, which will help to tone and strengthen the abdominal muscles.

DURATION

Beginner: The plow pose is not recommended for *Big Yoga* beginners.

Intermediate: Big Yogis are often very flexible by nature. If you fall into this category and have the strength to come into the plow with control, try doing up to three repetitions, only holding for a few breaths each.

CONSIDERATION

Be mindful of not forcing the feet to the floor and straining beyond your capacity. When there is extra weight in the belly, it can restrict breathing in this pose, causing discomfort. Thus, go at your own pace and do not exceed your own level of ease.

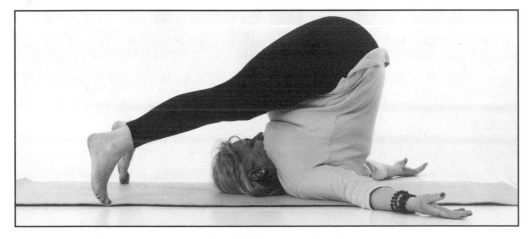

Lower the legs over the head in the Plow pose.

24. Fish

Matsyaansana

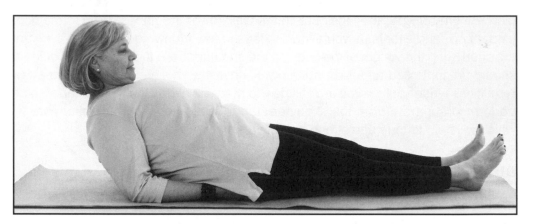

The first part of the Fish pose, with the head, neck, and shoulders off the ground.

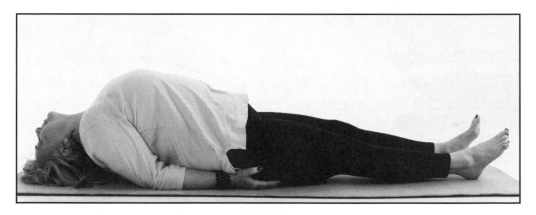

The second part of the Fish pose, with the back arched and the crown of the head on the floor.

BENEFIT

The fish pose is a counter pose to the shoulder stand (page 104), as it stretches the thyroid gland in the opposite direction, allowing the hormones to be released into the whole system. It also helps to correct posture problems and can improve asthmatic conditions. Stale carbon dioxide at the apex of the lungs is exhaled, and the whole capacity of the lungs is infused with fresh oxygen. In addition to giving a massage to the neck and shoulders, it strengthens the muscles of the waist, spine, and back.

TECHNIQUE

Begin in the supine corpse (page 62) with the feet together. Place the arms along-side the body and tuck the palms of the hands under the buttocks. Using the elbows and forearms for support, inhale and begin to raise up the head, neck, and chest until you are looking at your feet. Then, arch the upper body back on an exhale, al-lowing the crown of the head to come down to the floor. This should create a nice arch between the buttocks and the crown of the head. Feel the chest spread, have a little smile on the lips to relax the face, and breathe deeply. When coming out of this pose, inhale and raise the head, neck, shoulder blades, and chest up off the floor, so you are once again looking at your feet. Then, begin to release the curve of the spine and exhale down, vertebra by vertebra.

DURATION

Beginner: One round, held for up to three breaths, is sufficient.

Intermediate: One round, held for up to six breaths, is recommended.

CONSIDERATION

Be careful not to sneeze, swallow, or cough while doing the fish pose. Make sure you always come out of this pose by raising the head, neck, and chest completely off the floor, using the elbows for support. If you have a headache, refrain from doing this pose.

ADAPTATION

Use a bolster or a folded blanket under the shoulder blades for support, if needed.

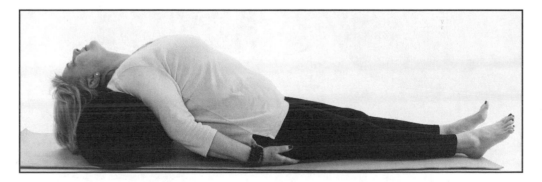

Fish pose adaptation using a bolster for support.

25. Bridge

Sethu Bandha Sarvangaasana

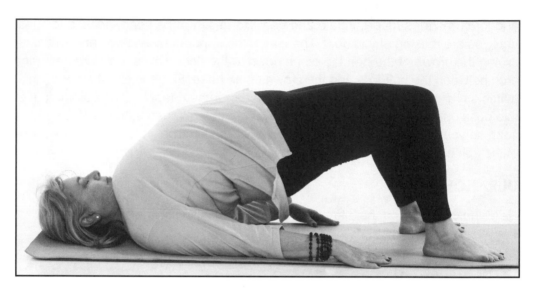

Bridge pose with the palms flat on the floor.

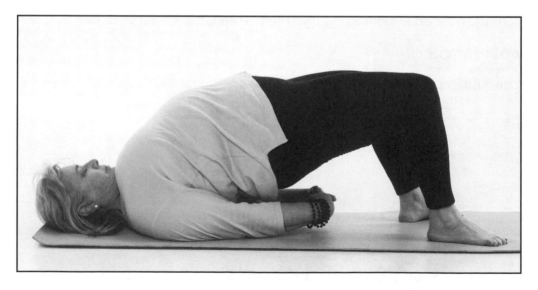

If you can interlace your fingers behind your back, go for it!

BENEFIT

The bridge pose strengthens the buttocks and hamstrings, opens the chest, and improves spinal flexibility. It also brings a fresh supply of blood to the pineal, pituitary, and thyroid glands, as well as to the head and neck.

TECHNIQUE

Begin in the supine corpse (page 62). Exhale and bend the knees, bringing the soles of the feet flat on the floor and sliding them close to the buttocks. Have the feet and knees hip-width apart. Inhale and begin to tuck the tailbone upward, lifting the hips up towards the ceiling. Bring the arms alongside the body, palms down, and roll the shoulders back and down. Lift the hips as high as you can while still remaining comfortable. Draw the chest toward the chin and hold the pose for a few deep breaths. To release, exhale and roll down, vertebra by vertebra, top to bottom, bringing the tailbone and buttocks down last. If you want to do another round, leave the knees up but relax the legs, letting the knees touch and rest a moment.

DURATION

Beginner: Do up to three rounds, holding each for up to three breaths.

Intermediate: Do up to three rounds, coming up a little higher with each round and holding the final round for up to six breaths.

CONSIDERATION

This pose is often taught with the arms straight and the fingers interlaced behind the back. If you carry your weight in the upper arms, though, it can be strenuous. That is why this version is offered. If your neck is stiff or weak, refrain from holding the pose and do a few shorter repetitions instead.

ADAPTATION

For a restorative variation, place a block, folded blanket, or bolster under the sacrum.

Twists

In this section, we're going to twist—but we're not going to shout! The various twists squeeze toxins from the spine, helping to keep it flexible and maintain its status as a good conduit for energy. The twists also massage and restore the adrenal glands—located on the backside of the body around the middle of the back—which are responsible for the "fight or flight" response. Coffee actually taxes these glands, so if you're a coffee drinker, these twists are very beneficial.

26. Half-Spinal Twist
    Arddha
    Matsyendraasana

28. Supine Twist
    Jathara
    Paarivartanasana

27. Easy Supine Twist
    Sumanas Jathara
    Paarivartanasana

26. Half-Spinal Twist
Arddha Matsyendraasana

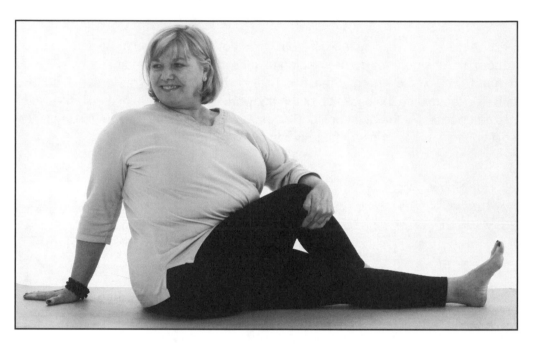

Twisting the spine from bottom to top in the Half-Spinal Twist position.

BENEFIT

In addition to keeping the spine flexible, the half-spinal twist massages the pancreas, assisting it in producing the proper amounts of insulin and digestive enzymes. Research has shown that Yoga can lower the need for insulin in diabetics, and the half-spinal twist may be the one pose that can assist in this process more than any other.

TECHNIQUE:

Begin by sitting on the floor and hugging the knees into the chest. Allow the breath to elongate the spine. Extend the left leg out in front of the body, in alignment with the left hip. Step over the outstretched left leg with the right foot (the right leg is still bent), placing it on the floor beside the left knee. Bring the right hand flat on the floor behind you, with the fingers pointing away from the body. Keep it close to the buttocks so that the arm stays perpendicular to the floor. Place the left hand on the top of the upraised right knee to use as a fulcrum to help you twist. Begin to turn on an exhalation, and look over the right shoulder, twisting the spine from bottom to top. Intensify the twist with each exhalation, but not beyond your capacity. Release the pose from top to bottom, beginning with the head and arms, and working your way down the spine. Repeat on the other side.

DURATION

Beginner: Perform this pose once on each side and hold for up to three breaths.

Intermediate: Again, once on each side is all that is needed, but hold the pose for up to six breaths.

CONSIDERATION

It's important to keep a lift in the spine so as not to crunch and injure the vertebra. Do your best to keep the spine perpendicular to the floor and not to tilt back. The closer the hand is to the buttocks, the easier this becomes. Come out of the twist as if you were moving through Jell-O, with fluid, rather than sudden or jerky motions, so as not to cause injury to the disks of the spine. Take care to keep the bottom of the chin parallel to the floor in order to keep the cervical vertebra in proper alignment. Keep the foot of the extended leg in line with the leg and hip, rather than flopping over to one side. All these instructions related to alignment are important, because when we move the body out of alignment, we are more apt to injure the disks in the spine, or to overstretch muscles that support us in this pose.

ADAPTATION

This twist can easily be performed sitting on a chair if you're not comfortable getting down on the floor. Sit facing forward in a chair with your feet firmly planted on the ground and your spine extended. Then, pretend you're at the movies and one of your friends sits down in the row behind you. Turn around to the right, grab the top of the chair with your left hand, and say hi! (No, don't throw popcorn!) Do another round on the opposite side. Another variation is to sit in any cross-legged position on the floor, ignoring the above instruction about having one leg extended and the other knee upraised. Simply bring one hand across the body to the opposite knee, place the other hand behind the back, close to the buttocks, for support, and twist.

27. Easy Supine Twist
Sumanas Jathara Paarivartanasana

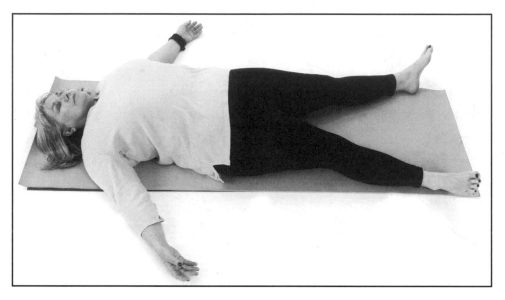

Begin on the back in the Supine Corpse.

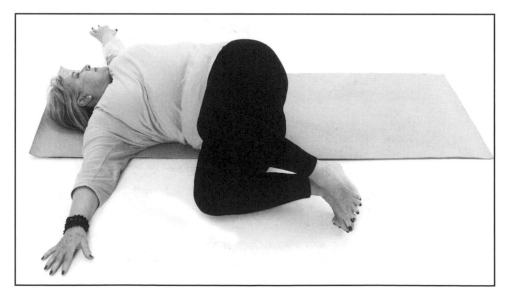

Bring both knees over to one side into the easy Supine Twist.

BENEFIT

The easy supine twist promotes flexibility of the spine. It is more relaxing than the half-spinal twist (page 116), which can be challenging to anyone carrying weight in the belly.

TECHNIQUE

Begin by lying on the back on the floor in the supine corpse. Extend the arms out to the sides, forming a "T" shape. On an exhale, draw the knees up to the chest and bring the arms in to hug them. Continue to breathe as you rock gently from side to side in order to create more space in the lower back area. When you feel comfortable, extend the arms again into a "T" shape, exhale, and lower both knees down toward the floor on the right side of the body. If the knees don't come all the way down to the floor, that's okay, simply stay in your comfort zone. To come out of the twist, inhale and bring the knees back to the chest. Repeat this same motion on the other side—dropping the knees to the left side of the body. This constitutes one round. In subsequent rounds, you can enhance the twist by adding a turn of the head in the opposite direction from the knees.

DURATION

Beginner: Hold for up to three deep breaths. I like to do anywhere from three to six rounds, but go at your own pace.

Intermediate: Hold the twist for up to six breaths and add the turn of the head. As you rest and hold the pose, feel the spine continue to release and extend. Three rounds are fine.

CONSIDERATION

Don't force the turn of the head, which could cause injury to the cervical vertebra.

ADAPTATION

If hugging the knees isn't comfortable, use a strap or tie to add a few inches for comfort.

28. Supine Twist
Jathara Paarivartanasana

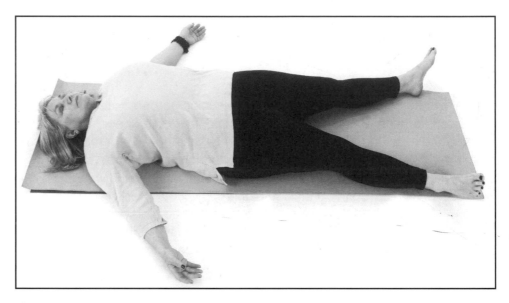

Begin on the back in the Supine Corpse.

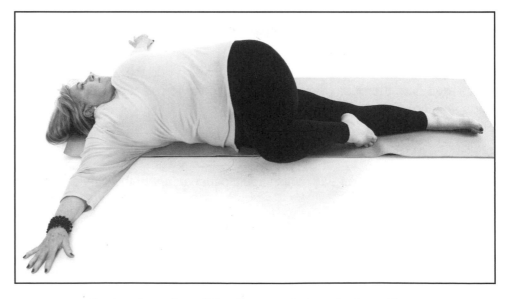

Finish with one knee "falling" over the body in the Supine Twist.

BENEFIT

Similar to the other twists, the supine twist beautifully opens the body. It tones the spine, exercises the lungs, and allows for a gentle, deep breathing practice.

TECHNIQUE

Lying on the floor in the supine corpse (page 62), bring the feet together and the arms out to the side in a "T" shape. Bend the knees as you slide the feet up toward the buttocks. Lift the buttocks, and with a deft adjustment, shift the right cheek over to where the left one was, without moving the torso. Extend the right leg so that it is aligned with the right hip, and place the sole of the left foot on top of the right knee. Leading with the left knee, allow the entire left side of the body to "fall" over to the right. Once you've reached the edge of your comfort zone, add a relaxed turn of the head in the opposite direction. For an added boost, draw the left knee down toward the floor with the gentle guidance of the right hand. Watch the effect of each inhalation and exhalation as you hold the pose. If you placed the hand on the knee, release it first, and follow by returning the head to the center. Then, bring the left knee and the rest of the body back to center to come back to the starting position, with the knees up and the hips back in alignment. For the opposite twist, begin by lifting the buttocks, placing the left cheek where the right one was, and continue.

DURATION

Beginner: One round, held for up to three breaths is sufficient.

Intermediate: One or two rounds, held for up to six breaths are fine.

CONSIDERATION

If you find your shoulder lifting on the opposite side from the direction of the twist, be aware of keeping it relaxed, as if it's melting down to the floor. It may not come to the floor, but soften it and allow it to release downward. Remember, we're trying to release tension, not create it!

Standing Poses

Standing poses are very popular in Yoga studios and gyms these days. They are the foundation of the *Vinyasa Flow*—a Yoga style in which a series of poses is performed in sequence with the breath. However, for a Big Yogi, doing standing poses for a long period of time can be hard on the feet, causing unnecessary discomfort. As soon as you feel any pain in the feet, it's time to move on to other poses that get you off of them. If you are regular in your practice, your feet will develop greater tolerance, but go at your own pace, especially if you are attending public classes. I would also caution you to be aware of the openness of the feet. Try to evenly distribute the weight of the body throughout the entire surface of the foot, and keep the toes long and wide.

29. Mountain Pose
    Tadaasana

30. King Dancer
    Natarajaasana

31. Warrior One
    Virabhadraasana One

32. Warrior Two
    Virabhadraasana Two

33. Triangle Pose
    Trikonaasana

34. Tree Pose
    Vrikshaasana

35. Intense Forward
    Stretch
    Uttanaasana

36. Stomach Lift
    Uddhiyana Bandha

37. Stomach Rolling
    Nauli Kriya

29. Mountain Pose
Tadaasana

BENEFIT

The mountain pose is the foundation for all of the standing poses. It improves posture, stability, and confidence.

TECHNIQUE

Stand with the feet parallel, about a hip-width apart. Stretch the toes upward, spreading them wide before allowing them to come back to the floor. Feel your weight evenly balanced throughout the surface of each foot. Soften and lengthen the back of the neck, but continue to lift from the base of the spine. Imagine that heaven has gravity, too, and is drawing you up. Throughout the exercise, keep the arms soft, hanging loosely alongside the body. Relax the shoulders but keep them wide, and lift up the breast bone as you breathe.

DURATION

Beginner: Hold for up to three breaths, as many times in your Yoga session as you like.

Intermediate: Hold for up to eight breaths, several times throughout your Yoga session.

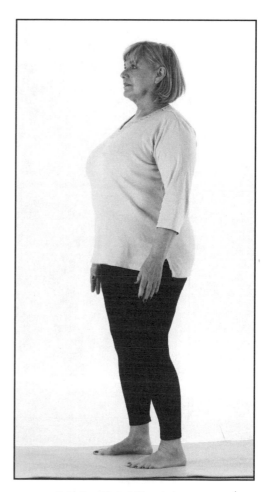

Standing in the Mountain pose.

CONSIDERATION

Carrying a lot of weight in the breasts can interfere with the ability of the shoulders and arms to relax, especially if you're wearing a heavy-duty bra with wires on the sides. If this is true for you, help the shoulders relax by drawing them gently up toward the ears and rotating them back, before releasing them down.

30. King Dancer

Natarajaasana

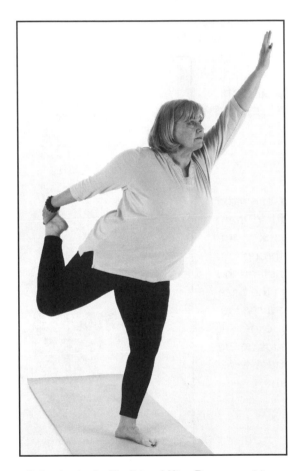

Balancing in the Traditional King Dancer position.

BENEFIT

The king dancer gives the spine, leg, and ankle muscles a good workout. It also improves posture and concentration.

TECHNIQUE

Begin by standing in the mountain pose (page 123), with the feet grounded into the earth and the eyes focused on a point in front of you. Bend the right leg back, and reach for the foot or ankle with the right hand. Raise the left arm overhead. Maintain your focus as you hold the pose, and feel the core of the body lengthening—lifting up and out of the hips. To come out of the pose, release the right leg from the right hand, and slowly return to the mountain pose. Repeat on the other side.

DURATION

Beginner: One or two rounds, held for up to three breaths, are fine.

Intermediate: If your balance is good, you can hold the pose once on each side for up to eight breaths.

ADAPTATION

Extra weight in the legs and torso can make it difficult to get the leg high enough for the hand to reach back and get a good grip. If you are experiencing this difficulty, try standing in a doorway, using the walls for support until you get into the pose. Alternatively, try standing next to a chair, using the back for support as demonstrated in the photographs below. Once you are in position and balanced, hold the pose, come out of it with control, and then switch sides. If you are still having trouble grasping the foot, use a strap, a tie, or a flip-flop to "lasso" the foot behind you.

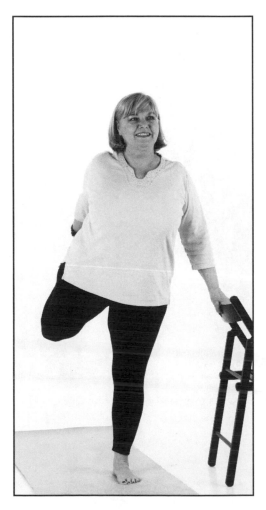

Coming into the pose using a chair for balance.

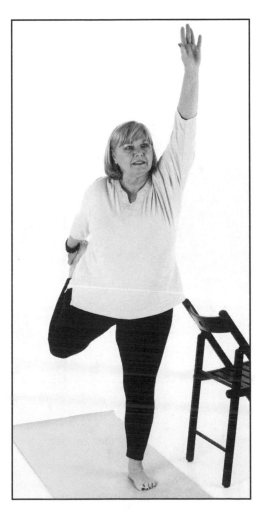

Balancing in the posture.

31. Warrior One

Virabhadraasana One

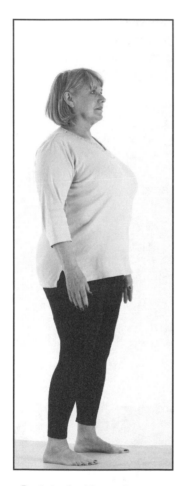

Begin in the Mountain pose.

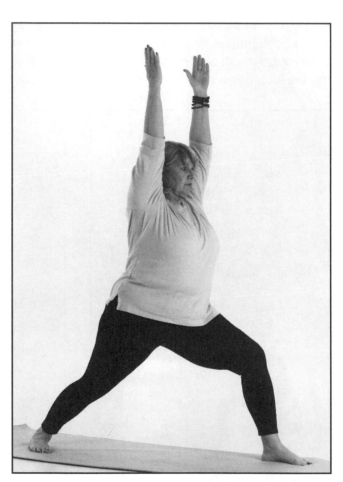

Raise the arms overhead into Warrior One.

BENEFIT

The warrior pose promotes confidence and strengthens the legs and ankles. It also stimulates the abdominal organs and gives a good stretch to the upper body. Additionally, this pose is therapeutic for flat feet, carpal tunnel syndrome, osteoporosis, and sciatica.

TECHNIQUE

Standing in the mountain pose, inhale and step the right foot a comfortable distance forward, up to three or four feet. Keep the outside of the right foot, which is now the front foot, parallel to the edge of the mat. Turn on the heel of the left foot—the back foot—so that the toes point away from the body at a 45 degree angle, keeping the leg straight and long. Square the hips forward in the direction of the right foot. Bend the right knee, bringing the top of the right thigh parallel to the floor if you can, and sink into the pose. Extend the arms out to the sides, palms up, and continue to raise them up overhead until they are perpendicular to the floor, in a "touchdown" position with the palms facing each other. See if you can perceive energy between the palms. Relax the shoulders away from the ears and engage the area at the bottom of the shoulder blades. To come out of the pose, rotate the arms out and away from each other so the palms face outward, and allow the arms to float down. Straighten the front knee, and begin turning to face the opposite direction so you can perform this pose on the other side. This constitutes one round. When you are done with both sides, come back to the mountain pose in reverse order.

DURATION

Beginner: One round, held for up to three breaths, is sufficient.

Intermediate: One round, held for up to six or eight breaths, is fine. You can always do more rounds if you enjoy it, though.

CONSIDERATION

Be observant of the feet. Try to connect the entire surface of the foot—especially the heel of the back foot—to the mat for best results.

ADAPTATION

If you feel unsteady in the initial stance, leave the arms down by the sides or bring them to the top of the bent thigh, until you gain more strength and balance.

32. Warrior Two

Virabhadraasana Two

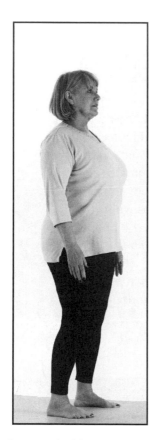

Begin in the Mountain pose.

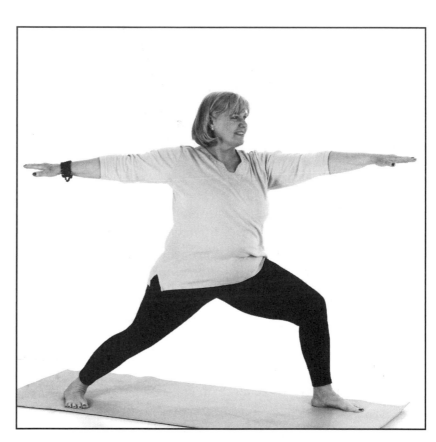

Inhale the arms up, parallel to the floor, into Warrior Two.

BENEFIT

Warrior two opens the shoulder joints and upper chest, thereby increasing lung function. It also tones the chest and upper-arm muscles, and increases blood flow and energy throughout the body.

TECHNIQUE

Standing in the mountain pose, inhale and step the right foot forward a comfortable distance, about three to four feet. Keep the outside of the right foot, which is now the front foot, parallel to the edge of the mat. Turn on the heel of the left foot—the back foot—so that the toes point away from the body a 45 degree angle, keeping the leg straight and long. Bend the right knee, bringing the top of the right thigh parallel to the floor if you can, and sink into the pose. Extend the right arm forward and the left arm backward, raising them up until they are at shoulder height, parallel to the floor. Look out over the fingers of the right hand and lengthen the arms. Imagine someone is gently pulling your fingertips in opposite directions. Keep the shoulders down and open. Feel that you are an invincible force in the universe. Release by straightening the front knee, allowing the arms to come back to the sides of the body, and returning the right foot to its starting position. Repeat on the other side.

DURATION

Beginner: One or two rounds, held for up to three breaths each, will begin to make you feel strong-like-bull!

Intermediate: One round, held for up to eight breaths, will make you feel invincible!

CONSIDERATION

Keep both feet flat on the floor for good balance and alignment, and imagine you are gathering earth energy through the feet. Don't allow the forward knee to extend past the foot, because doing so can compromise the knee joint and cause injury. Keep the arms parallel to the floor, thereby keeping them in correct alignment with the shoulders. If you find you are having trouble with balance, scoot the front foot sideways to widen your stance.

33. Triangle Pose
Trikonaasana

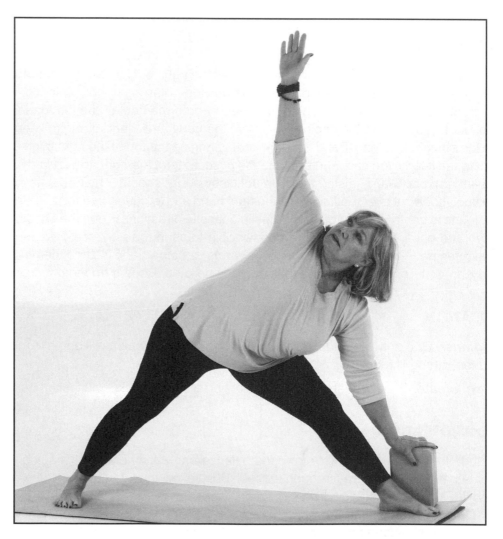

Bending sideways in the Triangle pose, using a block for support.

BENEFIT

The triangle pose tones the spinal nerves, diaphragm, and abdominal organs. It also tones the muscle fibers along the intestinal walls and increases peristalsis— the wave-like contractions that move food along the digestive tract. In addition, this pose tones the legs and strengthens the muscles and ligaments of the feet, thus providing more support for the larger body.

TECHNIQUE

Stand with the right foot in front of the left, in the same stance as the warrior poses (pages 126 and 128). Float the arms out to the sides until they are parallel to the floor at shoulder level, with the right palm facing down and the left palm facing up. From the waist, bend the trunk of the body sideways to the right, until the right hand reaches the right knee, shin, or foot. The left hip will move forward slightly. Keep the gaze upward toward the left palm, and breathe deeply. Inhale to come out of the pose, leading with the upraised arm, and sliding the right hand up the right leg for support, if necessary. When the torso is upright, lower the arms and bring the right foot back to the left. Take a few breaths before repeating on the other side.

DURATION

Beginner: One or two repetitions, held for up to three deep breaths, are recommended.

Intermediate: Hold the pose for up to six breaths. One round is all that's necessary.

CONSIDERATION

Take caution not to twist the knee out of alignment with the corresponding foot. On a personal note, I find this pose especially challenging because of the size of my prodigious belly. It prevents me from feeling the openness of the upper hip that I observe in my slender friends. Nevertheless, I still find benefit from triangle pose, and recommend it to all.

ADAPTATION

If it is uncomfortable to place the lower hand on the knee, shin, or foot, you can rest it on a block, a chair, or the thigh, instead. Additionally, the gaze can be forward instead of upward if that makes the pose more comfortable for you, but try to create and maintain space between the ears and the shoulder-tops, so as not to scrunch the neck. If you find your upper hip dropping forward, try doing the pose with your backside against a wall. This includes the head, shoulders, and the lower hip.

34. Tree Pose

Vrikshaasana

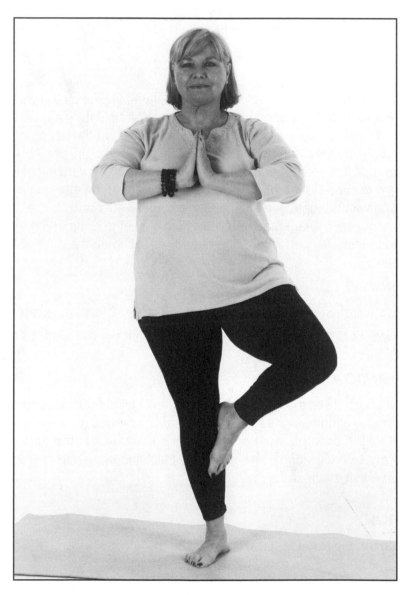

Balancing in the Tree pose with the hands
together in front of the chest in *anjali mudra*.

BENEFIT

The tree pose is a wonderful balancing pose that promotes self-confidence and strengthens the feet and legs.

TECHNIQUE

Standing in the mountain pose (page 123), bring all the weight onto the right leg. Bend the left knee and bring the left foot up to a comfortable place on the right leg. The left knee should be pointing out to the side, as if the legs were making the shape of the number four. When you are first beginning, only bring the left foot as high as the right ankle. When that becomes easy for you, move the foot up the leg toward the knee, or higher. Focus your eyes on a point in the space in front of you. Bring the hands together in front of the chest, in *anjali mudra,* which literally means "offering." When we perform it, we seal the energy from the palms into the heart center, creating a feeling of devotion. To come out of this pose, slowly lower the left foot back to the floor with control. Exhale the arms down and repeat on the other side.

DURATION

Beginner: Hold only as long as you can without falling. One or two rounds, held up to three or four breaths, are excellent.

Intermediate: One round, held up to five or six breaths, is fine. As you become steady in the pose, begin to raise the arms straight up overhead for a greater challenge, keeping the palms together.

CONSIDERATION

Be sure to have a chair, wall, or doorway to practice near, so that if you lose your balance you won't fall.

ADAPTATION

If you feel a little unsteady on your foot, stand next to a chair and perform the pose while holding the back of it with one hand, and raising the other up toward the ceiling.

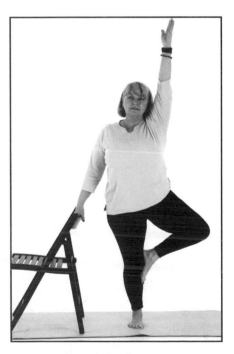

Tree pose adaptation
using a chair for balance.

35. Intense Forward Stretch

Uttanaasana

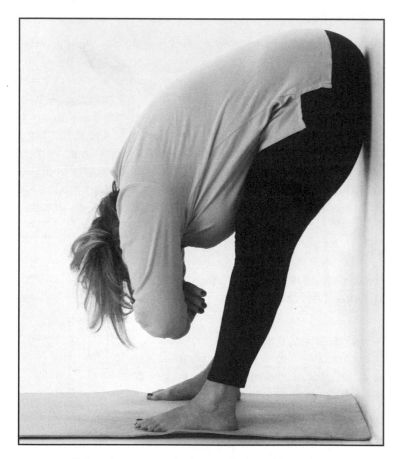

Fully released into the Intense Forward Stretch.

BENEFIT

Better than a coffee break, this stretch is a great antidote to hunching the shoulders forward while sitting at your desk. It reduces tension all along the spine and shoulders. Additionally, if you breathe deeply throughout the stretch, it can have profound effects on lowering the blood pressure.

TECHNIQUE

Begin in mountain pose (page 123) with the back, neck, head, and buttocks resting on a wall. Walk the feet about twelve to eighteen inches away from the wall, and spread them about a foot apart. Exhale and drop the chin to the chest. Keeping the buttocks pressed firmly against the wall, let the weight of the head carry your torso down slowly, deliberately rolling through each vertebrate in the spine. Stop anywhere along the way down to breathe deeply into any place that may be holding tension. Try drawing the belly up toward the spine at the end of the exhalations. Continue bending as far as you feel comfortable, keeping the legs soft or slightly bent—whichever feels best. The idea is to feel the "stretch" (actually it's a release) in the spine, as well as a strong connection to the earth through the feet and legs. To come back up, inhale, bend the knees a little more for support, and slowly roll up through the spine until the back, neck, and head are against the wall again. Pause for a moment. Gently shrug the shoulders up and back, and then release them. Feel the effects of this calming stretch.

DURATION

Beginner: It's not necessary to hold this pose longer than a breath or two. One round is sufficient.

Intermediate: Hold the pose for up to five breaths, and take your time rolling up and out of it. One round is sufficient.

CONSIDERATION

If you start to feel dizzy, slowly bring the head upright and look forward. If you're still feeling dizzy after a few moments, sit down and rest until you come back to normal. If you have sciatica, refrain from rolling all the way down to avoid aggravating your condition. Remember, honor your body.

ADAPTATION

If you need added support, place a chair in front of you and bring the arms to rest on top of the back of the chair. Continue to hold on as you roll down to keep yourself steady. See if you can create a little more space between the ears and the shoulders by softening and lengthening the neck.

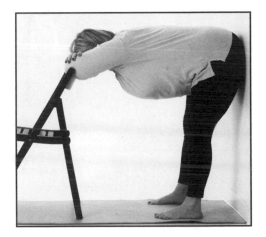

Intense Forward Stretch adaptation using a chair for support.

36. Stomach Lifts

Uddhyana Bandha

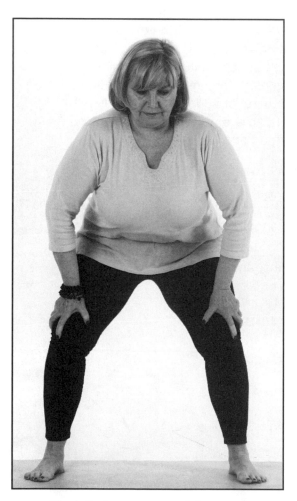

The belly drawn up toward the spine.

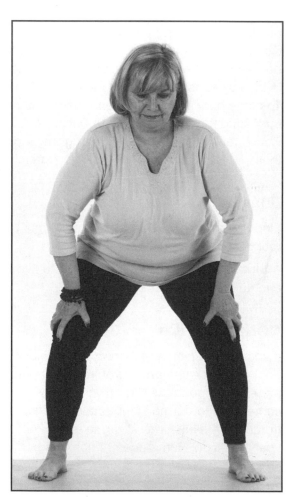

The belly pumped outward.

BENEFIT

Although a lock, or *bandha,* is not actually an asana, I am including *uddhiyana bandha* here because it is usually performed in a standing position. It is a wonderful tonic for the nerves of the solar plexus—the pit of the stomach. It also reduces abdominal fat, strengthens flabby stomachs, and relieves constipation, indigestion, and liver troubles. The ancient Yoga treatises even claim that this pose can conquer death!

TECHNIQUE

From the mountain pose (page 123), spread the feet about eighteen inches apart. Inhale, and then empty the lungs with a strong exhalation out of the mouth. Without inhaling again, bend forward slightly and place the hands on the knees for support. Continuing to avoid inhalation, draw the belly up toward the spine and maintain the lift. Before you feel the need to inhale, roll up and out of this position and begin to breath normally again. This constitutes one round of stomach lifts.

DURATION

Beginner: One to three rounds are good.

Intermediate: Three to five rounds are good.

CONSIDERATION

Care should be taken to not go beyond the capacity of the breath—don't wait till you're gasping for air to come out of the pose. Additionally, this pose is not recommended for people with serious abdominal troubles or circulatory disturbances.

ADAPTATION

After practicing this pose for some time, you can begin to pump the abdominal muscles—a purifying practice called agnisara, the fire dhauti. Begin as described above. After the exhale, draw the belly up toward the spine and pump it out and in using the muscles of the abdomen, until you feel the need to inhale. Then, roll up and out of the pose, and inhale with control.

37. Stomach Rolling
Nauli Kriya

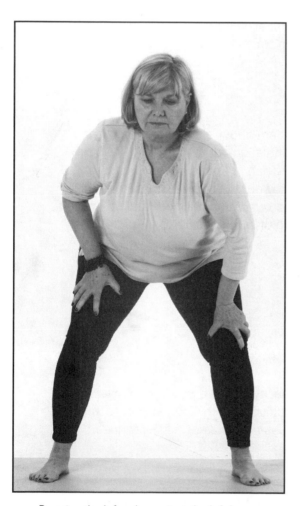

Pressing the left palm against the left knee.

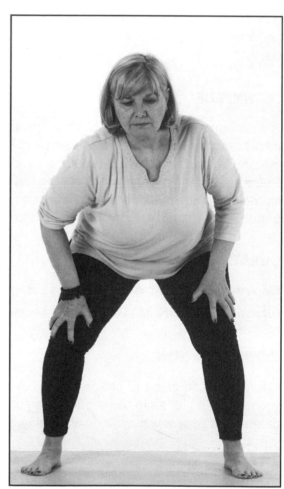

Pressing the right palm against the right knee.

BENEFIT

The stomach rolling pose benefits all the organs involved in digestion and regenerates the abdominal viscera, more commonly known as the "guts." For the Big Yogi, this pose helps to reduce abdominal fat and tone the belly. It's also beneficial in improving menstrual and fertility problems.

TECHNIQUE

From the mountain pose (page 123), bring the feet a little wider than hip-width apart. Inhale, and then empty the lungs with a strong exhalation out of the mouth. Without inhaling again, bend forward slightly, place the hands on the knees for support, and lift the stomach. With strong arms, begin to press the right palm against the right knee, followed by the left palm against the left knee. This will engage the muscles of the abdomen, or *abdominus rectus,* which includes the two bands of vertical muscles on either side of the belly button. When one side is engaged, the other side should be relaxed. Continue to alternate sides and repeat, remembering to come back to a full upright position before you inhale.

DURATION

Beginner: This exercise is not recommended for beginners.

Intermediate: Try doing three separate rounds, but only hold the breath for as long as is comfortable in each round.

CONSIDERATION

Stomach rolling is not recommended for people with high blood pressure, or who suffer from any abdominal illness. It should be practiced on an empty stomach. When constipated, have a cup or two of warm water before practicing it to help get the bowels moving.

ADAPTATION

Try having the heels of the feet close together with the toes pointed out. This may be a more effective stance for your body.

Seated Poses

Some of the following seated poses help to open the hips, work the muscles of the buttocks, and strengthen the back muscles that support the spine. Others are simply used as positions in which to work other parts of the body, including the shoulders, throat, and even the intestines! Ultimately, becoming comfortable in the seated poses will enable you to have a peaceful meditation, which is one of Yoga's higher goals.

38. Easy Sitting Pose
    Sukhaasana

42. Wind-Relieving Pose
    Pavanamuktaasana

39. Stick Pose
    Dandaasana0

43. Cow-Faced Pose
    Gomukhaasana

40. Bound Angle
    Baddha Konaasana

44. Lion Pose
    Simhaasana

41. Digestive Pose
    Vajraasana

38. Easy Sitting Pose
Sukhaasana

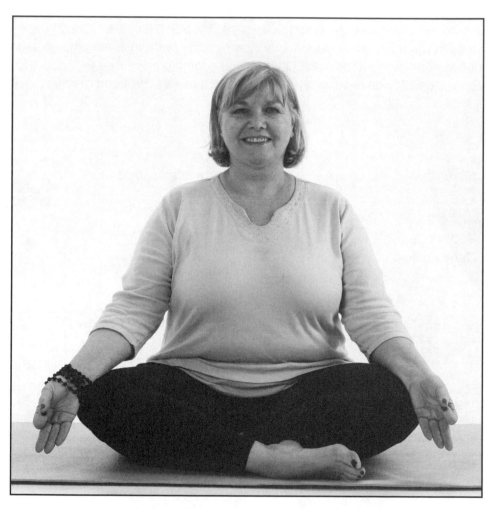

Seated with the legs crossed in the Easy Sitting pose.

BENEFIT

This easy sitting pose is a good preparation for more advanced sitting poses, which are used for meditation. It helps to open both the hips and inner thighs.

TECHNIQUE

This is the basic "criss-cross-applesauce" pose that children are taught in school. Begin by sitting on the floor with the legs extended in front of you. Rock a little from side to side or walk the hips back in order to achieve a firm connection between the sitting bones and the floor. Bend one leg then the other, bringing the feet to rest in front of the center of the body with the ankles crossed. Rest the hands on the knees, face up or face down—your choice. As you inhale, feel the chest expand and the spine lengthen. As you exhale, make any minor adjustments of the shoulders by rolling them up, back, and down. Close the eyes and mentally scan the body. Begin to observe the breath and relax.

DURATION

Beginner: Hold for two to five minutes, according to your capacity. See if you can keep your attention on the breath, but if not, watch where the mind goes and do your best to gently bring it back to the breath.

Intermediate: As you become more comfortable in this pose, you can hold it anywhere from five to thirty minutes as a meditation, which we'll learn more about beginning on page 179.

CONSIDERATION

If you are wearing a bra that has underwire, you'll want to adjust the position of your arms so you're not feeling compressed under the armpits.

ADAPTATION

If this pose causes discomfort in your knees, place pillows underneath them to provide added support. On the other hand, if your knees are high and having trouble relaxing downward, elevate the hips by placing a folded blanket or pillow under the buttocks. This should give the knees enough space to drop down. If you're using this pose for meditation, you may want to buy a meditation pillow, or *zafu,* which has a firm texture and gives good height, allowing the knees to open toward the floor.

39. Stick Pose

Dandaasana

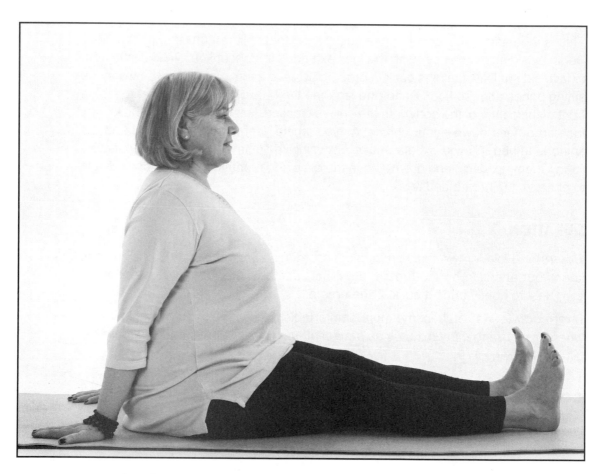

Lengthening the legs and spine, and lifting the chest in the Stick pose.

BENEFIT

The stick pose, as the name indicates, works the muscles of the back that support the "stick"—the spine. It also tones the abdominal muscles, the hip flexors, and the tops of the thighs. It is excellent preparation for other seated postures, as well.

TECHNIQUE

Sitting on the floor, extend the legs forward with the feet together. Place the hands behind the back, palms on the floor, with the fingers pointing away from the body. You may want to rock a little from side to side to release the sitting bones to the floor. Lengthen the legs and feel them extending through the heels. On the inhalations, lift the chest. On the exhalations, drop the shoulders and give them a little squeeze backwards—the back should be doing most of the work, not the arms.

DURATION

Beginner: Repeat throughout your Yoga session as a transitional pose anytime you're sitting, as many times as you like. Hold for up to three breaths.

Intermediate: Hold the pose for up to six breaths, and use anytime you like throughout your Yoga session.

CONSIDERATION

Be careful not to place too much pressure on the wrists. If you feel this happening, it is probably because you are using the arm muscles to prop you up, rather than engaging the back muscles. Also, if your belly creates an obstacle to keeping the feet together, open the legs a little wider.

ADAPTATION

If your wrists are delicate, try holding a block in each hand behind your back instead of placing the hands on the floor.

40. Bound Angle

Baddha Konaasana

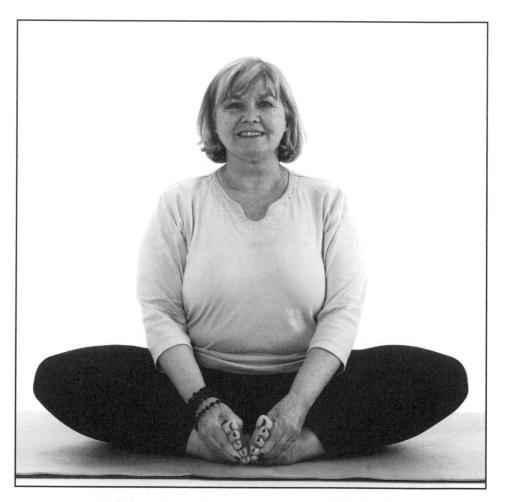

Relaxing the knees down toward the floor in the Bound Angle posture.

BENEFIT

The bound angle pose opens the hips, preparing the body for more challenging poses. It also frees and lengthens the lower spine. With practice, this pose becomes a comfortable, steady posture, suitable for meditation.

TECHNIQUE

Begin by sitting on the floor in the stick pose (page 144). Slowly bend the knees and draw the feet toward the body, bringing the bottoms of the feet together and allowing the knees to fall open toward the floor. As soon as you can reach them, take hold of the ankles with the hands and feel the chest expanding with deep inhalations. Squeeze the muscles of the outer hip, which will allow the knees to come closer to the floor, and then relax again. Experiment with the distance between the feet and perineum with two things in mind: keeping the spine long and lifted, and bringing the knees as close to the floor as possible.

DURATION

Beginner: Hold the pose for up to three breaths and repeat if you like.

Intermediate: Hold the pose from three to six breaths and repeat if you like, although one round is sufficient.

CONSIDERATION

If you carry your weight in your thighs, your knees may become stressed in this pose. If you are experiencing any discomfort, try rotating the flesh of the upper thighs outward. Or, try sliding the feet a little farther away from the torso.

ADAPTATION

If having both knees bent is uncomfortable, try bending only one leg at a time. If it's difficult to keep the spine lifted, place a folded blanket or pillow under the buttocks.

41. Digestive Pose
Vajraasana

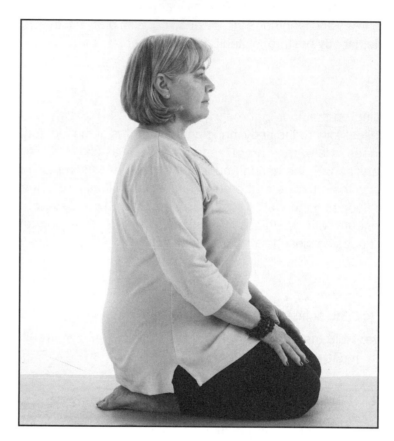

Kneeling on the ground in the Digestive pose.

BENEFIT

This pose aligns the digestive organs, which helps speed up the digestion process, making it an ideal pose for after Thanksgiving dinner—before the pie! It tones the thighs and legs, and relieves gas, indigestion, and sciatica, as well. Alternately, this pose is called *vajraasana*—the heroic pose—because it gives a sensation of self-confidence. The chest, and therefore, the heart, is opened up during this pose. When you are able to hold it for longer periods of time, it becomes a stable pose, suitable for breathing exercises and meditation.

TECHNIQUE

Kneel on the ground, keeping both the knees and the feet together. Bring the buttocks down to rest on the feet. You can separate the ankles, but keep the toes together. Let the hands come to rest on top of the thighs, with the palms facing down. Lift upward through the spine, but keep the shoulders relaxed and down. Keep the breath soft and even throughout.

DURATION

Beginner: One or two rounds, held only as long as you are comfortable, are good. Because it's not a position we Westerners are accustomed to, it may not be comfortable to hold for very long. Don't overdo it! Improvement will come over time, with practice.

Intermediate: One round, held up to six breaths, would be sufficient. The more frequently you practice this pose—even throughout your day or while you are watching television—the more beneficial it will be.

CONSIDERATION

Many people have trouble with the flexibility of their knees. If you find that this pose makes you uncomfortable, try out one of the many adaptations. Do not force your body into a position for which it is not ready.

ADAPTATION

If your knees are giving your trouble, try placing a folded blanket or pillow either between the thighs or behind the knees, under the buttocks. If it is the ankles, not the knees, that are bothering you, try placing the folded blanket or pillow under the shins, from the knees down to the ankles. If you're still miserable—and many people are—you can try using a meditation bench (see page 185), which gets the weight off the ankles and offers a lesser stretch to the knees. If none of these options work and you still aren't comfortable, bring the hands to the floor in front of you and lean the body forward to relieve pressure. Over time, your ability to get comfortable in the traditional digestive pose will improve, and it's definitely worth it!

42. Wind-Relieving Pose

Pavanamuktaasana

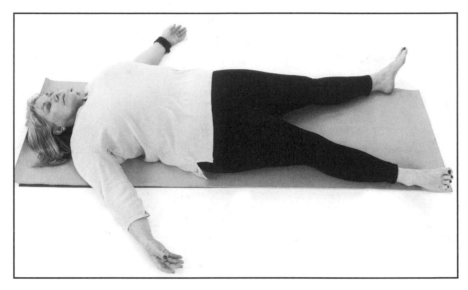

Begin on the back in the Supine Corpse.

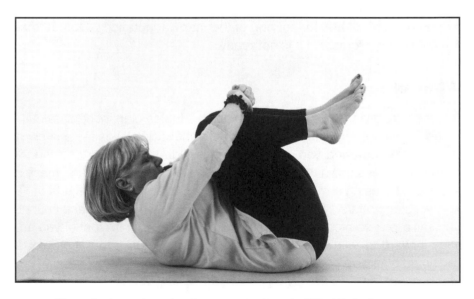

Draw the knees into the chest to come into the Wind-Relieving pose.

BENEFIT

This pose is an excellent tonic for digestive problems. It increases peristalsis—the movement of food through the digestive tract—and allows excess gas to be expelled. Additionally, it can be beneficial in releasing pain from the lower back, and can adjust minor misalignments, as well. The wind-relieving pose also gives a good stretch to the buttocks.

TECHNIQUE

The wind-relieving pose isn't really a seated pose, but directly after the digestive pose seemed like the best place to include it! Resting on the back in the supine corpse, exhale and draw the knees up toward the chest. Grasp the shins with the hands and continue to breathe. As you exhale, give the belly a good squeeze, drawing it down toward the spine. Don't be surprised if you pass a little gas. If you would like a deeper stretch, lift the head, bringing the chin toward the chest as you continue to hold the pose. Be sure to keep breathing, relaxing on the inhale and compressing the belly on the exhale. After the suggested number of breaths, gently release the legs and bring the entire body back to the resting pose.

DURATION

Beginner: One or two rounds, held up to three or four breaths, will be fine.

Intermediate: One or two rounds, held for three to six breaths, will be fine.

ADAPTATION

If the belly poses an obstacle to grasping the shins, use a strap or tie to create an extension.

43. Cow-Faced Pose
Gomukhaasana

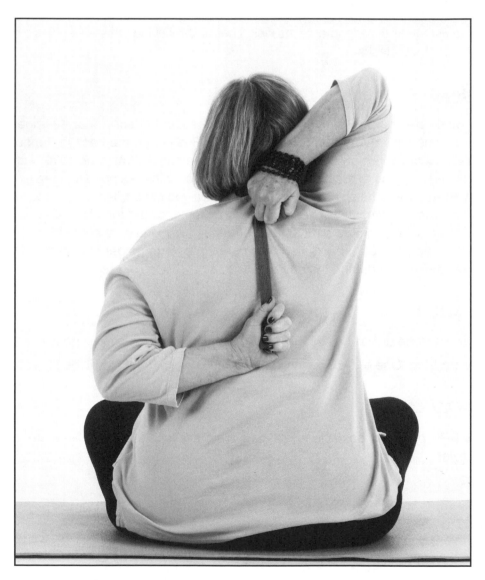

Stretching the arms and chest in the Cow-Faced pose,
using a strap to create extension.

BENEFIT

The cow-faced pose is excellent for relieving general stiffness in the upper chest, shoulders, and neck. It also stimulates the kidneys, alleviates tiredness and anxiety, and is a good tonic for adult-onset diabetes.

TECHNIQUE

In any comfortable, seated position, place the left hand on the lower back with the palm facing out. Raise the right arm overhead, bend the elbow, and with the right palm facing the spine, reach for the fingers of the left hand. If you can bring the raised elbow behind the head, you can exert a gentle pressure on the arm with the head to get good extension. Close the eyes and relax the neck. Begin to exhale out of the pose in reverse order, and repeat on the other side. This constitutes one round.

DURATION

Beginner: One or two rounds, held up to three breaths, are sufficient.

Intermediate: One or two rounds, held up to six breaths, are sufficient.

CONSIDERATION

If you feel constricted in this pose, it could just be your bra! Try wearing one without underwire, or let the girls completely loose.

ADAPTATION

If you aren't able to reach the opposite hand, use a strap or tie to create extension.

44. Lion Pose

Simhasaasana

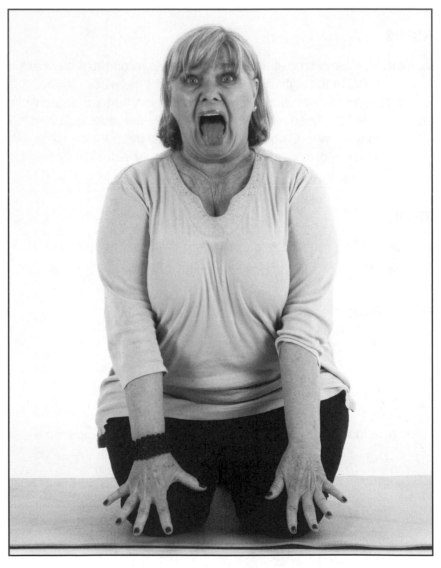

Tensing the entire body, especially the throat area, in the Lion pose.

BENEFIT

The lion pose is beneficial for the throat, and is therefore especially good for singers and those who speak publicly. It also brings energy to the eyes, ears, and nose, and soothes tension in the chest and diaphragm.

TECHNIQUE

Sitting in the digestive pose (page 148), bring the hands to the knees with the fingers spread apart. Exhale and draw the belly toward the spine. All at once, tense the whole body. Stretch out the arms and fingers, raise the eyebrows, and stick out the tongue. You can also cross your eyes and focus at the space between the eyebrows. Then, inhale and relax.

DURATION

Beginner: Only hold as long as the exhalation. Repeat up to three rounds.

Intermediate: Only hold as long as the exhalation. Repeat up to five rounds.

ADAPTATION

The toes of the feet can be flexed for an even sturdier stance. If you're not comfortable in the digestive pose, though, simply try sitting in any comfortable, seated position.

Chapter 6

Breathing Practices

Every time you finish practicing Yoga's physical postures, it's important to spend a little time re-oxygenating the blood through the practice of Yogic breathing, or *pranayama*. During the physical poses—through the stretching and squeezing of the muscles, organs, and glands—toxins are driven to the bloodstream for elimination. Breathing techniques, then, will refresh the blood and energize the whole system. The benefits of breathing practices are gained during the inhalations, when fresh energy is deliberately brought into the body, and also during exhalations, which should always be smooth, quiet, slow, and controlled. And although it's a subtle practice, it's very powerful.

Personally, I love pranayama. I'm a singer and a swimmer, so I think I was born to love breathing. Once, I heard Frank Sinatra talking about his singing technique. He said the reason he had such exquisite vocal control and could sing long phrases without breathing, was because he used to practice holding his breath in a swimming pool in Vegas. He would take a deep breath and swim the entire length of the pool without coming up for air. In a way, he was practicing pranayama, which loosely translated, means breath (*prana*) control (*yama*).

> "Breath is the bridge which connects life to consciousness, which unites your body to your thoughts."
>
> THICH NHAT HANH

Actually, *prana* is more than breath. It literally means the life force of the universe, akin to "chi" or "ki" in the Asian traditions. Hawaiians call it "nama," Egyptians called it "ka," and in *Star Wars*, Yoda called it "the force." Regardless of the name, however, it always refers to the vital energy that causes any kind of motion, down to the smallest atom. We imbibe this life force from the food we eat, the water we drink, the air we breathe, and the sun that shines down on us. As we breathe, oxygen enters our lungs and its energy gets infused into our bloodstreams. This sends pranic energy into every cell of our bodies, charging us up with new vitality. (I've even read that prana goes *in between* each cell!) Yoga will train you to actually perceive this energy as it enters your body, and teach you to begin to control it. Once you can control the prana in your own body and mind, you can begin controlling the universal prana, as well.

THE ELEMENTS OF PRANAYAMA

There are three major elements to pranayama: exhalation (*rechaka*), inhalation (*puraka*), and retention (*kumbhaka*). Another, more advanced component of pranayama is suspension of the breath. When the breath comes to rest automatically, without effort, it is called *kevala kumbhaka,* and it is then that you will experience the beautiful stillness of the prana mentally, physically, and energetically. This state builds subtle power and enables the body to burn up impurities in the system.

A personal experience of mine provides a great example of this. I grew up back in the day when smoking was "cool" (hard to imagine, now). Both of my parents smoked, and as soon as I went to college I started smoking, thinking it made me appear sophisticated. I continued to dabble in smoking for a few years before I started studying Yoga. After I had been studying Yoga seriously for about a year, though, I caught a bad respiratory infection—complete with a sore throat and headache—that prevented me from smoking. Instead, I drank a lot of pure, fresh juices and kept doing my Yoga and pranayama exercises. When I was finally over the cold, I found I no longer had any desire to smoke! Smoking gave *me* up! The nicotine had been purged out of my body. What a gift!

THE BENEFITS OF PRANAYAMA

Approximately 5,000 years ago, Patanjali wrote in the *Yoga Sutras* that by engaging in the practice of pranayama, "The veil over the inner light is destroyed." This supreme inner light to which he referred is in each of us and is a common theme in all major religions. Unfortunately, in most of us it is covered by a veil of mental darkness. But by the regulation and restraint of the prana, and its ability to make both the mind and body move, the mind is able to come into stillness and the inner light is uncovered.

To put it simply, Yogis believe if we can control the breath, we can control the mind. Try to remember the last time you were working on something that required your full concentration. After some time, without being aware of it, your breath probably stopped! Then, unconsciously, you took a little gasp of air to get the breath going again. This is because when the mind becomes focused on one thing, the breath slows way down. Conversely, when we are excited or upset, the breath becomes quick and irregular. If we consciously slow the breath down, though, the mind will follow and become quiet and focused. Hence, controlling the breath allows us to control the mind.

"The goal is to know yourself. The way is to clean up the mind."
SRI SWAMI SATCHIDANANDA

Additionally, pranayama purifies the nervous system and makes the body light and the mind alert. It also promotes a good appetite and aids digestion. Moreover, in spring and fall when allergens abound, a regular pranayama practice can alleviate allergies and asthma. In winter, it can prevent colds and flus by strengthening the immune system. And in summer, there are even practices that can cool the body.

The Five Subtle Bodies

The ancient Yoga texts describe five sheaths, or bodies through which the human being functions. The physical body, or *Anna Maya Kosha,* is the most obvious. It is the dimension of the organs, blood, bones, and skin. Subtler than that is the body of energy, the *Prana Maya Kosha,* which incorporates the vital force that keeps the physical body healthy. Subtler still is the body of will, the *Mano Maya Kosha.* It is the dimension linked to the subconscious mind, and includes our mental abilities, knowledge, and perception, as well as our psychological state—namely, our feelings about things.

Next, we find the dimension of higher wisdom, the *Vijnana Maya Kosha.* This sheath is where our wisdom and our ability to differentiate right from wrong reside. And finally, the subtlest, yet most powerful sheath is the body of bliss, the *Ananda Maya Kosha.* We become aware of it when we have a peaceful moment of joy, such as when we experience a beautiful sunset or awake from a restful night's sleep.

In working with the Yoga asanas, we first tune into the physical body. Gradually, through our regular practice, we become more established in connecting with the more subtle bodies. In pranayama, we are learning to regulate pranic energy, which in turn gives us the ability to regulate the thoughts in the mind at the body of will level.

Breathing Techniques

There are several different breathing techniques in Yoga. Before you begin practicing them, though, take a minute to evaluate your breath as it is now. Do you inhale and exhale through your nose or mouth? The following Yogic breathing techniques should always be done with the mouth closed, unless otherwise noted. If you currently breathe through the mouth while it is open, this will take some getting used to.

Additionally, observe how your stomach moves when you breathe. Most new students are so conditioned to hold their stomachs in to appear thinner, that they have developed into reverse breathers. In other words, instead of expanding the belly on the inhalation, they hold it in. And instead of pulling the belly in on the exhalation, they push it out. This style of breathing prevents the lungs from expanding and sacrifices a wellspring of energy that could be available in every breath. So, when doing the following breathing exercises, focus on breathing in and out through the nose, as well as on expanding the belly during inhalations, and allowing it to contract during exhalations.

45. Simple Three-Part Breath

Deergha Swasam

BENEFIT

The simple three-part breath is the foundation of all the breathing practices. When agitated or upset, it can calm the mind. Conversely, when drowsy or sluggish, it can perk you up by bringing fresh energy into the system. It also helps to clear the blood of toxins after your Yoga practice. When fully expanded, the lungs can hold up to seven times as much air as in normal breathing, and more air means more *prana*—more vitality and more joy! The three parts of the breathing capacity are the abdomen, the rib cage/middle chest, and the upper chest. In the simple three-part breath, we work up to the point where we are filling all three with air and prana.

TECHNIQUE

Begin by sitting in a comfortable position, either cross-legged on the floor, or in a chair with the feet grounded about a foot apart. Elongate the back, widen the shoulders, and relax the rib cage downward. Close the eyes and begin to watch the breath. The action of the belly should be expansion on the inhale—the way a balloon expands when you fill it up with air—and contraction on the exhale, as if you had let all the air out of a balloon.

As a way of learning how to do all three parts of this breath, we'll first do one section at a time. When you are ready to begin, take a breath and fill up the belly, feeling it expand. Then, exhale slowly, quietly, and with control. Repeat this a few more times, keeping the focus on just the belly. Once you have mastered that, take a breath and fill up both the belly and the rib cage with air, expanding the breath from the bottom of the lungs upwards. Exhale first from the rib cage, then from the belly. Again, repeat this action a few times. Finally, take a breath and fill up the belly, rib cage, and the upper chest with air. You may feel the collarbones rise slightly, but don't let the shoulders creep up. Now the lungs are fully expanded. The exhalation starts at the top of the lungs, goes through the mid-section, and finally, the bottom of the lungs empties as the belly collapses and is drawn in toward the spine. When you have filled the lungs completely and exhaled fully, you have completed one round. Once you have an awareness of all three parts, this practice becomes a continuous flow of breath, in and out.

DURATION

Beginner: Start by focusing on only filling the belly, making sure to allow it to puff out a little bit. Then, build on that by filling the rib cage and upper chest. Exhale in reverse order, and repeat for up to three rounds.

Intermediate: Once you reach full lung expansion—abdomen, rib cage, and upper chest—continue in the slow, deep breathing for a while, up to ten rounds. To bring more awareness to your practice, begin to count the inhalations and exhalations. Work toward making the exhalations at least as long as the inhalations, and eventually, up to twice as long.

CONSIDERATION

If you find that your belly is going in on the inhale and out on the exhale, you might be doing reverse breathing. To retrain your body and change your breathing habits, try doing the three-part breath while lying on your back on the floor. Place one hand on the abdomen, below the belly-button, to monitor the movement of the breath. Observe the expansion on the inhale and the soft collapse on the exhale. Spend some time enjoying the gentle rise and fall of the belly, and before long, this type of breathing will become natural for you.

46. Hissing Breath
Ujjayi

BENEFIT

In Yogic breathing, the longer the exhalation, the more benefit you gain, as the prana remains in the body longer. One way to slow down the exhalation is to use the hissing breath. When used in a meditative state, this breathing technique calms the mind and gives a good focal point for restless thoughts. The hissing breath also brings good circulation to the throat and is helpful in relieving sore throats. Additionally, it is said to improve digestion and respiratory problems, and to bring a luster to the face.

"May today there be peace within.
May you trust God that you are exactly
where you are meant to be.
May you not forget the infinite possibilities
that are born of faith.
May you use those gifts that you have received,
and pass on the love that has been given to you.
May you be content knowing you are a child of God.
Let this presence settle into our bones, and allow your soul
the freedom to sing, dance, praise and love.
It is there for each and every one of you."
ST. THERESA

TECHNIQUE

As a stand-alone practice, the hissing breath can be done in any comfortable sitting position. Begin by partially closing the glottis muscles at the back of the throat, just behind the larynx. The glottis is a combination of fleshy folds and the space between the folds. It has the ability to open and close, creating different vocal sounds. When completely closed, it creates the "frog" sound. When partially closed, it creates the distinctive sound of the "H" in Hanukkah. The result of breathing while the glottis is partially closed will be a soft, hissing sound every time you take a breath. The friction this creates generates heat in the body. Therefore, it is widely used in some schools of Yoga throughout the asana practice, to enhance the burning of toxins in the system.

DURATION

Beginner: The hissing breath is not recommended for beginners.

Intermediate: The hissing breath can be used throughout your asana practice, according to your own capacity. In your pranayama session, use it to control the exhalations, making them up to twice as long as the inhalations. Do up to eight rounds.

CONSIDERATION

Do not to strain the throat. To avoid doing so, slowly build up to a longer practice over time.

47. Skull Shining Breath

Kapalabhati

BENEFIT

This technique helps purify the nerve centers in the skull—the *naadis.* It is also known as the "breath of fire." Personally, I like to think of the skull shining breath as "mental floss," as it helps to give you a clear head. It is also helpful in removing impurities from the bloodstream, as well as for warming up and energizing the body.

TECHNIQUE

Sitting in any comfortable, steady position, begin with a long, deep inhalation, followed by a slow exhalation—use the same three part breathing technique as in the

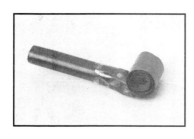

Party Squawker

simple three-part breath (page 162). Next, draw a short inhalation into the belly, and then quickly and sharply force out, drawing the abdomen up and in toward the spine. (This short exhale from the belly requires the same force used to blow the nose, so be sure to have a tissue handy just in case!) When you relax the belly, the breath will immediately want to come back into the body, so allow that to happen naturally. Repeat this action several times (check the duration below for specifics) before finishing with a long, deep inhale and a slow exhale. This constitutes one round. Because the skull shining breath is stimulating, it is good to follow it with the nerve purifying breath (page 168), which is gentle and calming.

DURATION

Beginner: Repeat the pumping action approximately ten to twenty times each round. Three rounds are recommended.

Intermediate: Repeat the pumping action approximately twenty to forty times each round. Three rounds are recommended, and they can be repeated at different times during the day.

CONSIDERATION

If you begin to feel dizzy, please stop and take a break. You can try again later if you wish, but don't overdo it. If you have high blood pressure, please refrain from practicing the skull shining breath unless you have the permission of your doctor. Also, if you are pregnant or in the midst of your menstrual cycle, this practice is not recommended. And finally, post-partum mothers should wait a few months before resuming this breathing technique.

ADAPTATION

If you are having trouble, try out one of the following tricks I've picked up both during my own practice, and through the observation of my students. First, if you're having trouble with reverse breathing (drawing the belly in toward the spine on the inhale, rather than letting it expand), go out and purchase a party squawker—the little things you blow into at birthday parties that make a loud, duck noise. It's almost impossible to blow into one repeatedly without correctly engaging the abdomen. Another trick is to slow down the skull shining breath, so that you are deliberately forcing the air in before pushing it out. Often, when we slow things down we can better understand the mechanics of how things work, and then build on that awareness over time.

48. Nerve Purifying Breath

Naadi Suddhi

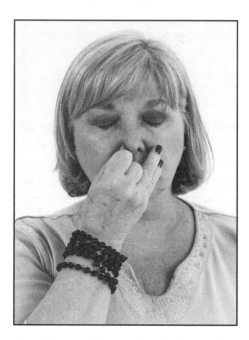

Closing the right nostril with the thumb.

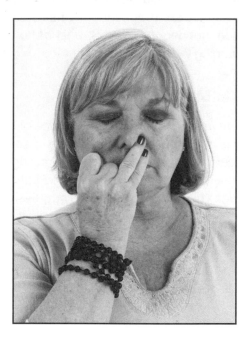

Closing the left nostril with the last two fingers.

BENEFIT

The nerve purifying breath calms the mind, soothes the nervous system, improves digestion, and helps with sleep disorders. It is a gentle breath that balances the right and left brain, and it is especially appropriate before meditation. *Naadi* is the Sanskrit word for nerve—but not in the Western sense of the word. There are 72,000 naadis that originate in the spine; however, we are mainly concerned with the fourteen main naadis—similar to the meridians used in acupuncture—which are channels that carry blood, water, and vital fluids throughout the body. Although we usually think of the naadis as being in the physical body, they have their counterparts in the subtle bodies, as well (see page 159). Bringing prana into the subtle bodies through the practice of the nerve purifying breath becomes a powerful force for transformation.

TECHNIQUE

The nerve purifying breath—also known as the alternate nostril breath—uses a *mudra,* or seal, called Vishnu mudra. (Vishnu is one of the Hindu gods, known as the preserver the universe.) Sit cross-legged or in any comfortable, steady position, with the spine long and the shoulders wide. To make Vishnu mudra, make a gentle fist with the right hand, then extend the thumb and the last two fingers. Keep the index and middle fingers tucked into the fleshy pad at the base of the thumb. Bend the right elbow, keeping the arm close to the chest, and bring the hand up toward the nose. After taking a full breath through both nostrils, close off the right nostril with the thumb, and exhale through the left nostril. Keep the right nostril blocked as you inhale through the left nostril, using the simple three-part breath (page 162). After a full inhalation, close off the left nostril with the last two fingers and release your thumb from the right nostril so you can exhale through the right side. Continue in this pattern, always switching nostrils after the inhalation, ending with a final exhalation on the right side. Bring the hands to the lap and take a moment to feel the peaceful effect of the practice.

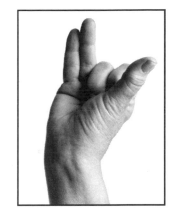

Vishnu mudra

As you get the hang of this pranayama, begin to count your inhalations and exhalations, using an "om" between numbers: "Om one, om two, om three, om four, om five . . ." After a few cycles, see what the average ratio is. Initially, you want the exhalation time to equal the inhalation time. With regular practice, you may find that the exhalations begin to lengthen naturally. Increase the length of the exhalations until they are up to twice as long as the inhalations.

DURATION

Beginner: Beginners can practice the nerve purifying breath for up to three minutes, finishing with the last exhalation on the right side.

Intermediate: As your exhalations become twice as long as your inhalations, you can begin increasing the number of repetitions, according to your capacity. When you are able to do several rounds comfortably, you are ready for the more advanced practice of the nerve purifying breath with retention (page 170).

CONSIDERATION

Make sure there is no strain in the lengthening of the exhales. Keep the breath slow and steady throughout. In addition, every time you switch to the opposite side, keep the breath soft, with no jerking.

49. Nerve Purifying Breath with Retention

Sukha Purvaka

BENEFIT

After you have practiced the traditional nerve purifying breath for some time and have developed the capacity to do ten rounds with the exhalations twice as long as the inhalations, you may begin to add the retention of breath. The retention of the breath enriches the blood and purifies the nerves throughout the body, which has a calming effect. At the same time, holding the pranic energy in the body longer creates amazing vitality and resistance to disease.

TECHNIQUE

Sit in any comfortable meditative pose. Begin with a full, deep breath through both nostrils. Making Vishnu mudra with the right hand (see pages 168 and 169), close off the right nostril with the thumb and exhale through the left nostril. Inhale into the left nostril and hold the breath as you gently drop the chin to the chest, into *jalandra bandha*—the chin lock. Gently contract the glottis (see page 162) to hold the air in the lungs, and remove the right hand from the nose, allowing it to rest on either the heart or the knee, whichever is more comfortable. Keep the mind focused on the energy in the spine, or on some peaceful thought or mantra. Before you feel the need to inhale, raise the head up and gently release the glottis. Bring the right hand back up to the nose and, making Vishnu mudra, close off the left nostril with the last two fingers. Exhale through the right nostril. There might be a slight pause in the breath at the end of the exhalation—that's natural. Then begin again, this time inhaling into the right side, holding the breath, and exhaling out of the left side. This constitutes one round.

DURATION

Beginner: This is not recommended for beginners.

Intermediate: Only hold the breath a short time, beginning with a ratio of ten counts on the inhalation, ten counts on the retention, and twenty counts on the exhalation. Continue alternating in this way for several rounds and finish with meditation. Over time, with regular practice, you can increase the retention, but consult a professional Yoga teacher before you do.

CONSIDERATION

Avoid even the slightest strain, and never hurry this breath. It's important to realize how subtle the power of pranayama is, especially when using more advanced techniques like the retention of breath. In the ancient Yoga scriptures, the power of prana is likened to a dangerous cobra. When we know how to control it, we can be like a snake charmer, and make the cobra dance. However, if we try to play with the cobra without proper preparation or training, it can kill us! If you are practicing retention of the breath, you should be avoiding alcohol, drugs, meat, and other stimulants, and living a pure, disciplined, Yogic lifestyle. Otherwise, Swami Satchidananda warned that pranayama could disturb the system, and even upset the mind to the point of insanity.

ADAPTATION

After you've practiced this breath regularly for a few months, you can also add *moola bandha,* the anal lock, which again, helps to seal energy into the body. On the inhale, draw the anal sphincter muscles up, tightening them into a secure seal, and hold as you hold your breath. Release moola bandha and jalandra bandha simultaneously, with control, as you exhale at the end of a round.

50. Bellows Breath with Chin Lock

Bastrika with Jalandra Bandha

BENEFIT

The bellows breath promotes healthy lung function by reducing phlegm and mucus, thereby making it a helpful exercise for those with allergies or asthma. It also helps to heat up the body and purify the blood.

TECHNIQUE

The bellows breath uses the same technique as the skull shining breath (page 166), with the addition of breath retention. After the first round of forced exhalations, make a long deep inhalation and hold the breath while dropping the chin to the chest into *jalandra bandha*—the chin lock. Hold the breath gently and repeat a mantra or embrace a beautiful thought, as your pranayama practice will give your mind power. When you are ready, bring the head up slowly and exhale deeply, with control. Imagine having a little lift, or slight inhalation, before you begin to exhale, which will release the glottis. Don't allow the breath to explode into the exhalation—no sound of grunting should be heard. Remember that it takes time to raise the head and exhale, so plan ahead and don't hold the breath too long—you don't want to be gasping for air.

DURATION

Beginner: This is not recommended for beginners.

Intermediate: If you have a regular pranayama practice, begin experimenting with the rentention of breath, using the ratio of ten counts for the inhalation, ten counts for the retention, and twenty counts for the exhalation. Moola bandha, the anal lock, (page 171) can also be added after several months of regular practice.

CONSIDERATION

This practice isn't for beginners. You should not begin experimenting with retention until you've been practicing pranayama regularly for a few months. If you begin to feel dizzy, please stop and take a break. You can try again later if you wish, but don't overdo it. If you have high blood pressure, please refrain from practicing the skull shining breath unless you have the permission of your doctor. Also, if you are pregnant or in the midst of your menstrual cycle, this practice is not recommended. And finally, post-partum mothers should wait a few months before resuming this breathing technique.

A Word about Nasal Cleansing

A practice called *water neti* or *water jala,* can be used to prevent colds and clean the nasal passages. You can get a little neti pot at your local health food store. When you get it home, fill it with warm water and add salt—about a half teaspoon of salt per cup of water. Lean over the sink and turn the head to the side. Pour the saltwater into the upper nostril and let it run out the lower nostril. Do a few rounds of neti on that side, and then move to the other side. If you don't have a neti pot, you can simply put the salty water in the palm of your hand or in a glass, and gently snuff the water up the nostril. This practice is especially helpful in keeping the sinuses clear when you have allergies or a cold.

---

51. Cooling Breath
Sitali

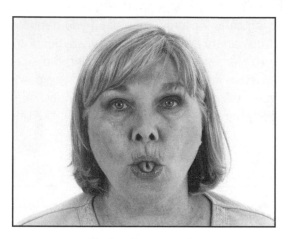

Curling the tongue in
preparation for the Cooling Breath.

BENEFIT

The cooling breath helps remove heat from the body—both heat from other Yoga practices and heat from the weather. It also reduces hunger, thirst, and sleepiness. In my long drives from my home in Michigan to the Yogaville Ashram in Virginia, I have often used this exercise to wake me up at the wheel when I feel a little drowsy. It really works!

TECHNIQUE

Sit in a comfortable meditative position, with the spine long and the shoulders wide. Begin with a complete exhalation through the nose. Then, curl the sides of the tongue up and in, lengthwise. Stick the newly shaped tongue slightly out of the mouth and wrap the lips around it. This creates a "straw," which will cool the air as it enters the body. Inhale deeply through your "straw," and then draw the tongue in and close the mouth. Hold the breath for a few seconds as you focus on the cooling sensation in the body, before closing the mouth and slowly exhaling through both nostrils.

DURATION

Beginner: Three to five rounds are sufficient.

Intermediate: Three to eight rounds are sufficient.

ADAPTATION

Not everyone can curl their tongues into straws. If you are one of the people that can't, replace the cooling breath with the wheezing breath (page 178), which is a pranayama that has similar benefits.

52. Humming Bee Breath
Bhramari

BENEFIT

The humming bee breath is great for the vocal chords and it promotes a good night's sleep. It also provides a real experience of the bliss of the primordial hum of the universe—*pranava ananda.* This hum, which is in everything as the vibrating life force, is a nearly imperceptible sound that is suitable for meditation. Because of its subtlety, we make an approximation of it by humming. This makes an easy focal point for a peaceful meditation, as the mind can continue to "hear" the humming long after you have finished.

TECHNIQUE

Sitting comfortably in a meditative pose, close the eyes and inhale completely, through the nostrils. On the exhalation, close the lips and make a humming sound. Be aware of the buzzing of the bones in the cranium. Imagine the vibrations going straight up through the crown of the head and out into the universe.

DURATION

Beginner: Do five rounds at various pitches.

Intermediate: Again, five rounds at various pitches are sufficient.

53. Humming Bee Breath with Six-Way Seal

Bhramari with Shanmuki Mudra

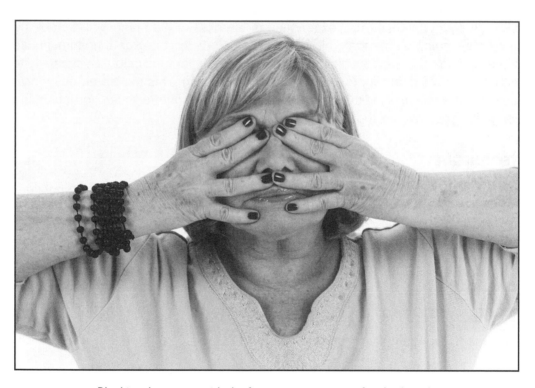

Blocking the senses with the fingers in preparation for this breath.

BENEFIT

Adding the six-way seal to the humming bee breath enhances its benefits, because it shuts out external noises and draws the awareness deeper within.

TECHNIQUE

This pranayama uses the same technique as the humming bee breath (page 175), only this time, all the senses are blocked. In preparation, sit comfortably and close your eyes softly. Raise the arms in front of you, palm ups, until they are parallel to the floor. Then, bend the elbows, bringing the hands toward the face. Plug the ears with the thumbs, lightly cover the closed eyes with the index and middle fingers, and spread the last two fingers downward, so that the ring finger is resting above the lips (be careful not to block the nostrils) and the pinky finger is resting below the lips. In addition, contract the muscles of the anal sphincter in *moola bandha,* the anal lock. Inhale completely, through the nostrils. On the exhalation, close the lips and make a humming sound—all the while keeping the senses blocked.

DURATION

Beginner: This pose is not recommended for beginners.

Intermediate: Hold the breath only as long as is comfortable, according to your capacity. As you exhale, release the anal lock but keep the hands in place for the next round. Do five to eight rounds at different pitches, and then take some time for a deep and serene meditation.

CONSIDERATION

Be careful not to press the eyelids too hard—the fingers should simply rest on them. This is a very advanced practice. Please wait until you have mastered the traditional Yoga postures and the nerve purifying breath (page 168) before trying the six-way seal.

54. Wheezing Breath
Sitkari

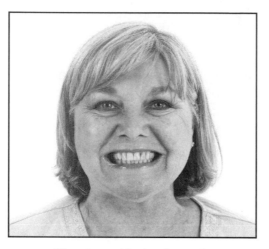

Clamping and baring the teeth
in preparation for this breath.

BENEFIT

The wheezing breath cools the body and keeps the gums healthy.

TECHNIQUE

Sit comfortably in a steady posture with the spine long and the shoulders wide. Begin by gently clamping and baring the teeth, as if you were smiling through clenched teeth. Then, curl the tongue back so that it touches the soft palate at the roof of the mouth, and inhale through the teeth, making a sucking sound. You will feel a coolness as the air enters the sides of the mouth. When you have inhaled completely, hold the breath a few seconds and focus on the cool sensation in the gums and tongue. Then, exhale slowly and deeply.

DURATION

Beginner: A few repetitions are fine.

Intermediate: Five to eight repetitions are fine.

Chapter 7

Meditation

Simply put, meditation is the process of bringing the mind to focus on one thought or idea, uninterrupted, for a long period of time. Normally, the mind is consumed with the normal chatter we are all familiar with. Sometimes it is useful, such as when we're planning events or accomplishing specific tasks, but other times it becomes obsessive-compulsive nattering. Quieting this incessant flow of thought is a slow process that requires the discipline of a world-class athlete, a will of steel, and a heart of pure gold. Luckily, the practices of classical Yoga are here to help you. Before we jump right into meditation, however, let's go back and take a look at our tree of Yoga.

THE TREE OF YOGA

As the sage Patanjali discusses in the ancient text, the *Yoga Sutras,* there are eight limbs on the virtual Yoga tree. These limbs spell out the basic habits a Yogi needs to practice in order to gain mastery over the mind, body, and senses. When mastery is achieved, the Yogi attains the highest goal—realization of the True Self. The limbs of the tree are as follows:

1. Self-Restraint (*Yama*)
2. Observances (*Niyama*)
3. Poses (*Asana*)
4. Breath Control (*Pranayama*)

5. Sense Withdrawal (*Pratyahara*)
6. Concentration (*Dharana*)
7. Meditation (*Dhyana*)
8. Self-Realization (*Samadhi*)

The first four limbs of the tree of Yoga aren't necessarily sequential. It's hard to determine where one practice ends and another begins. In other words, it's not as if you must practice and perfect self-restraint before moving on to observances. The physical poses—Hatha Yoga—are generally known as Yoga's

A Little Bit of Yoga Philosophy

As previously mentioned, the great sage Maharishi Patanjali compiled decades of previously unwritten Yogic wisdom in his classic text, the *Yoga Sutras*. He wrote about an eight-limbed tree of Yoga, describing the various practices that allow the Yogi to transcend the body and mind in order to achieve the ultimate goal of Yoga: Realization of the True Self. Hatha Yoga is what most people envision when they think about Yoga, but there are actually two limbs that come before it on the Yoga tree: Yama and Niyama. So, let's take a minute to learn about them.

Often called the Ten Commandments of Yoga, Yama and Niyama set forth basic rules of conduct that are helpful in keeping the mind and body clean and calm. Based on ethical and moral perfection and control of the senses, Yama and Niyama make us better humans. Remember, however, that these are simply guidelines for your own benefit. My guru, Swami Satchidananda, never said, "Don't do this, or don't do that." He used the analogy that a doctor would never send a sick patient away, telling him to get well, and then come back for treatment! The regular practice of Yoga is a cure-all and can help you drop bad habits naturally. There's never any need to force it.

YAMA

Yama, the Sanskrit word for restraint, includes five simple behaviors to avoid as you deepen your commitment to a Yogic lifestyle:

- *Non-violence (Ahimsa).* This can be interpreted as non-killing, as well as restraining anger. A fit of anger causes a reaction in the physical body, causing the endocrine system to pour out hormones that upset the body's natural harmony. St. Francis wrote, "Make me a channel of your peace." You may be familiar with pictures of him, surrounded by all the little animals. They had no fear of him because he was established in non-violence, and around him all hostilities and fear ceased to exist. Strive to be the same.

- *Truthfulness (Satya).* When we tell the truth, we never have to worry that someone is going to catch us in a lie. This helps keep the mind peaceful, which also has a calming effect on all of the subtle systems in the body.

- *Non-stealing (Asteya).* Stealing creates negative karma—for the victim and the thief. In addition, the act of stealing affects the mind, and subsequently, the body.

- *Continence (Brahmacharya).* This means self-restraint or moderation in all things, specifically sex. Not because there's something wrong with sex, but because it can become a distraction to the goal of Yoga. Anything that we can easily become attached to is gradually jettisoned in order to attain the higher goal. This helps build, rather than dissipate, energy.

- *Non-greed (Aparigraha).* This is the concept of not hoarding. Yoga is all about flow. If we come from a mind-set of lack and feel we have to hold on to things, we may gather physical clutter, which will ultimately clutter our minds, as well.

NIYAMA

There are five simple *Niyamas*—observances or practices—that are recommended:

● *Purity (Saucha)*. This involves keeping the body clean from the outside, and keeping the diet clean, as well. We even include purity of the thoughts, and refrain from unkind or vulgar thinking.

● *Contentment (Santosha)*. Accept life on life's terms, without resistance. When the resistance comes, we challenge ourselves to watch it, rather than to give into the battle. This is really living your Yoga.

● *Austerity (Tapas)*. This is the practice of accepting, but not causing pain. Jesus touched on the same idea when he spoke about turning the other cheek. It is said that accepting pain that comes to you, especially when you feel you aren't deserving of it, helps to burn up karma and purify the ego.

● *Spiritual Study (Svadhyaya)*. On the days when I just can't seem to get my body on the mat, I find solace and comfort by reading an uplifting book. Time and again, I find myself going back to my guru's teachings, but there are thousands of good books on Yoga, meditation, Buddhism, spirituality, and the like, available today. Check out the resource section (page 209) for books that may inspire you.

● *Surrender (Ishwarapranidhana)*. The final observance is surrender, or devotion. The ancient *Yoga Sutras* translates *Ishwarapranidhana* to mean, "Self-surrender to the Lord." And who is the Lord? The Supreme Consciousness that wakes you up every morning and makes the physical body function in thousands of ways, without any effort on your part. You can call it God, Higher Power, or whatever you feel comfortable with. When we surrender to that Higher Power, we become an instrument in the hands of the Divine. My friend Christine calls it, "Riding the horse in the direction it's going."

Practicing the Yamas and Niyamas will help to preserve and maintain your energy. One of the ancient Sanskrit *slokas*, or prayers, says, "May we gain energy to know the truth." If we're sickly or neurotic, how can we achieve anything? It is said that if you practice these ten basic principals, you will be leading an exemplary life. You will exude a natural joy and charisma, and you may begin to find that everyone will want to be your friend!

"calling card," and most people are first drawn to this third limb. It may be some time before they are even aware of the first two limbs, and that's okay.

As we continue to climb higher, we learn about the ever more challenging aspects of bringing the senses under our control, which will in turn teach us to control our minds. In a way, all the practices taken from the tree of Yoga that we have learned about so far, prepare us for meditation. The *yamas* and *niyamas* prepare us morally and ethically to lead a life of purity and contentment. The *asanas* improve the health of the body and make us fit for sitting comfortably for longer periods of time. The *pranayama* practices restore clarity to the mind, calm the nerves, and fill the body with energy.

Now, we're ready to take on something more subtle, more challenging, and ultimately, more rewarding. Gradually, all these practices will begin to merge, and you will find yourself moving from one to another as you explore different aspects. As Yoga Master B.K.S. Iyengar declared, "All the eight limbs of Yoga have their place within the practice of Yoga."

THE FIFTH LIMB—SENSE WITHDRAWAL *(PRATYAHARA)*

Before we can attempt to have a successful meditation (the seventh limb on the Yoga tree), we must first settle the mind by controlling sensory input—a practice known as sense withdrawal, or *pratyahara*. Pratyahara is the fifth limb on the Yoga tree, and it is loosely translated from Sanskrit to mean, "turning the senses inward." So, instead of allowing our senses to go out into the world and gather information for our minds to organize and assimilate, we turn them inward. Without the stimulus of the sensory input, the mind becomes clear and calm. And when the mind is calm, it reflects the true nature within, which is exquisite peace and bliss.

Don't get me wrong, this is not to say our senses are bad! Their job is to bring information into the mind so that we can function in our everyday world, and this is a good thing! Just imagine what it would be like to lose even one of your senses for a day. Take your sense of touch. Could you text your friends without being able to feel the keyboard? Could you play your guitar? Could you avoid burning your fingers when preparing a meal? Without sensory input from our skin, our days would certainly be difficult.

At the same time, however, when the senses are undisciplined, they just keep bringing more and more input into the mind, which can make us a little nutty—especially since the explosion of new media. How many social networking accounts do you have now? Are you on Facebook, Twitter, Myspace? How many times a day are you distracted by your emails? Personally, I know that if I spend too much time in front of the computer, I'm likely to fall down the rabbit hole like Alice in Wonderland. And then there's the phone. Many people have more than one phone number, making us way too easy to get in touch with. And that's not even mentioning texting!

To put it simply, our minds are constantly barraged with input from our senses, putting us on "overwhelm." It's no wonder that more and more people are being diagnosed with sleep disorders. Thankfully, Yoga has techniques to calm and soothe the overwhelmed mind. These techniques teach us to move our awareness away from the external world, and instead, focus it within. They also encourage us to turn off the radio, dim the lights, and close our eyes. Ahhh, I feel better already . . .

When we practice sense withdrawal, we gain control over the senses and can disconnect them at will from the sights, sounds, smells, tastes, and feelings of the external world—similar to a tortoise contracting his head and limbs. We accomplish this by using our discriminative faculties, which say to the mind, "Yes, that ice cream really looks tasty, but I have a lunch date in an hour and if I eat it, I'll spoil my appetite." We then redirect the mind to something elevating, and become absorbed in that instead.

Desires from memories of pleasurable experiences distract and disturb our minds. In the case of the ice cream, once we have enjoyed it we want to experience that yummy feeling again and again. Sense withdrawal, or *pratyahara*, allows the intelligence of the mind to gain control over these memories, though. So, instead of letting the memory of a delicious ice cream experience trick us into an act of impulse, the intelligence, or discriminative part of the mind puts on the brakes, draws the awareness back inside, and enjoys the contentment of the undisturbed mind.

If you have taken a Yoga class already, you may have noticed how your asana practice naturally draws your senses inward, giving you a deeper experience of your inner self. If you're really paying close attention to the body during an asana, your senses will automatically be put on temporary hold, and you won't even notice the smells of a delicious lunch being prepared in the kitchen, for instance. This is similar to artists, who become oblivious to extraneous noises in their environments when they're hard at work creating sculptures, poems, or songs. And how often have you heard someone say to their partner, who is engrossed in reading the morning paper, "Have you actually heard anything I said?" This is all sense withdrawal at work.

THE SIXTH AND SEVENTH LIMBS— CONCENTRATION *(DHARANA)* AND MEDITATION *(DHYANA)*

After learning to calm the mind by bringing the senses under your control, you can begin to sit for meditation. Your beginning meditations will essentially be an attempt at concentration—called *dharana* in Sanskrit. *Dharana* is the sixth limb on the Yoga tree, and it is the process of bringing the mind back to focus on your chosen object of meditation whenever it wanders. Later in this chapter, you will be given some suggestions as to what you can concentrate on.

True meditation, or *dhyana*, occurs when there is a continuous flow of uninterrupted thought onto one point. It has been likened to the flow of oil from the pitcher, the stream of oil, and the vessel receiving the oil. There is no break in the flow. With more experience, this will begin to happen naturally and spontaneously if you're regular in your "sitting" practice. Sri Patanjali says in the *Yoga Sutras* that you have to practice "for a long time, without break, and with all earnestness." For ease of description throughout this book, when I refer to meditation, I am referring to both of the sixth and seventh limbs on the Yoga tree—concentration and meditation.

THE EIGHTH AND FINAL LIMB— SELF-REALIZATION (*SAMADHI*)

When meditation is perfected, it leads to the experience of *samadhi*, or liberation. This is an experience of total bliss and peace. Self-realization is the eighth limb on the tree of Yoga, and is the ultimate goal of all our practices. Yet, since it is an experience that is beyond the mind and senses, it is very difficult to discuss. Therefore, I will simply say that it is just something you have to experience for yourself. You will know it when it comes, and I promise it will be worth the effort!

OVERALL BENEFITS OF MEDITATION

According to recent studies, the brain is capable of thinking 600 thoughts a minute! These thoughts, or *vrittis*, are usually in complete control of determining our experience of life, because we identify with them and tend to think they are all true. In reality, however, this is delusion. Our minds are so cluttered that our thoughts get intertwined, and they obviously aren't all true!

The process of watching the mind through meditation helps it to clear itself, sort of like defragmenting a computer's hard-drive. When the hard-drive is clean, the computer runs more efficiently and with fewer glitches. Similarly, when the mind is calm, the essential peace at the core of your being is tangible. During meditation, powerful forces that are stored up in the unconscious get released and raise themselves up to the conscious and subconscious levels. Mental clarity and balance are restored. Even subtle changes in the body can occur, healing it at the energetic level for a greater sense of grounding and ease.

According to the National Center for Complementary and Alternative Medicine (part of the United States National Institutes of Health), regular meditation can improve longevity and quality of life. One study found that meditation had the ability to reduce blood pressure by as much as 10 millimeters of mercury (mm/Hg) systolic (the top number), and 6 mm/Hg diastolic (the bottom number). In another, participants in an eight-week mindfulness meditation course experienced a decrease in negative emotions, which were still measurable long after the study was over! These same participants also showed a better immune response—when given flu vaccines, they produced more antibodies than people who did not participate in the meditation course.

Additionally, as science continues to study Yoga, it becomes increasingly clear that meditation can be a key component in reversing heart disease. A regular meditation practice helps to lower blood pressure, heart rate, and the stress hormones, which can also be a factor in weight gain. It also reduces the risk of heart attack, stroke, and atherosclerosis. And that's only scratching the surface of meditation's benefits!

In the workplace, meditation can improve productivity and reduce healthcare costs. For allergy sufferers, meditation can assist the body in boosting the immune system, making it less prone to attack. Like allergies, cancer is an auto-immune disorder, and meditation has been proven to decrease the chance of recurrence in cancer survivors. Furthermore, when we meditate regularly we gain a greater awareness of troublesome habits and mischievousness mind tricks, making it a useful tool in weight-loss programs, as well. And ultimately, meditation creates a feeling of inner peace, boosts mood, and helps to dispel the illusion of separateness.

PREPARING TO SIT FOR MEDITATION

As with any endeavor, meditation takes some preparation. Compare getting ready to sit for meditation to getting ready to go to sleep at night. Most of us have a ritual that prepares us for sleep. We change into our pajamas, wash our faces, brush our teeth, set our alarms, and fluff up our pillows just the way we like them. We might have a cup of hot tea and spend some quiet time reading, as well. All of these preparations signal our minds that we are about to take our rest. Here are some similar things to be aware of when getting ready to meditate:

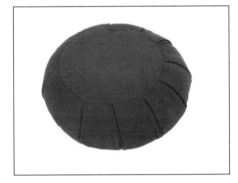
Zafu

Sitting Position

Of all the many tips that can help you prepare for a peaceful meditation session, perhaps the most important is to have a comfortable seat. Try sitting cross-legged on the floor, using a pillow under the buttocks. There are special meditation pillows, called *zafus*, which are specially designed to support a comfortable sitting position for the meditator. Or, you might want to try a slanted meditation bench. These take the weight off the knees, and also create excellent

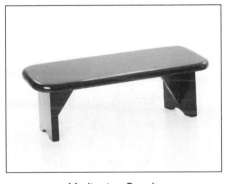
Meditation Bench

alignment and an openness in the spine. Both of these items are readily available. See the resource information at the back of the book (page 212) for more information.

Another option is to sit in a straight-back chair, taking care to keep the spine long and the shoulders wide, which allows the energy to flow upward to the higher energy centers. The most important thing is to find an easy position that you can maintain for the duration of your meditation. Make a vow, or *sankalpa*, that you are not going to move a single muscle until you finish. If possible, sit facing North or East, because aligning the body with the energy of the earth and its poles will have a beneficial effect.

Clothing

During meditation, wear loose clothing that doesn't restrict your breathing. It is helpful to do some breathing exercises before you begin meditating to stimulate the nervous system and re-oxygenate the blood, and as you're breathing deeply, you don't want be thinking about how tight your pants are. Also, since the body will cool down as you relax deeper into meditation, you may want to have a sweater or shawl nearby in case you get chilly.

Time of Day

The best time of day to meditate is at dawn, before the commotion of the day sets in. According to Ayurveda—the companion science to Yoga and the oldest known science of India—the hours between two and six in the morning are the hours of mental clarity, which makes them a suitable time for meditation. If you have a hard time waking up early and find yourself dozing during meditation, try doing a few asanas before you start. You might also try splashing some cold water on your face, taking a cool shower, or having a cup of tea to help get your mind alert. Another good time of day to meditate is right before bedtime, as meditation helps calm the mind so you can have a peaceful night's sleep. But ultimately, the best time of day to meditate is whatever time you will do it regularly! A regular meditation practice at a certain time of day that fits well in your schedule is far greater than a sporadic practice at dawn.

Empty Stomach

If you are meditating in the morning, try to have your elimination before you begin. In the evening, wait a few hours after dinner before your meditation. Don't meditate on a full stomach. When you are digesting food your blood goes directly to your stomach, making you want to take a nap. As the stomach is empty, feel that the eyes are empty, too—not flitting back and forth in rapid eye movements. Keep them soft and closed: the awareness is inward, and the eyes are at rest. If you find the eyes are having a trouble settling down, try a few rounds of the eye exercises, beginning on page 47.

Length of Meditation

When you begin to practice, try to sit for ten or fifteen minutes, twice a day. Then, as you become more comfortable, you can gradually increase the time you set aside for your meditation. It's better to be regular with two short meditations every day, than to meditate for an hour once a week. The most important thing, though, is to listen to your body and be kind to yourself.

Attitude

Meditation brings us into the element of the sacred, and should therefore be approached with reverence. Chanting "om" three times will help bring your mind to focus and give it the idea that it is time to settle down. If you're not comfortable with the sound "om," you can use a familiar sound from your own tradition, such as "Alleluia," "Amen," or "Allah." (Isn't it interesting how similar these words sound?) Then, recite a prayer or affirmation of your own, or begin to learn the Sanskrit prayers, or *slokas*, provided on page 190.

Training the undisciplined mind is similar to training a puppy, and both require patience and compassion. When we are training a puppy, we give it signals to let it know when it's time for different activities, and when it runs away, we gently call it back. Similarly, we offer the chanting at the beginning of meditation so the mind knows it's time to settle down. And if the mind wanders during the meditation, we gently but firmly bring it back to the object of meditation, which we'll discuss later. Then, at the end of meditation, we again chant "om" three times to let the mind know the meditation time is over, which will leave it refreshed and happy.

Breath

As you meditate, tune into your breath. When it comes into the body, feel it going right through your spinal column down to the base of the spine, and then observe it return upward through the crown of the head when you exhale. This, in itself, is a profound meditation. Alternatively, simply listen to the sound of the breath. Even though that sounds easy, you might be surprised at how many times the mind will want to think about something else!

Progress, Not Perfection

Tend to the process of meditation, rather than the goal. Remember, meditation is a science! If you do it with good intention, you will get good results.

MEDITATION TECHNIQUES YOU CAN TRY

There is no "right" way to meditate. There are as many different types of meditation as there are people meditating. And every time you meditate, it will be a fresh, new experience. However, I want to give you some suggestions for different meditation techniques. They come from a variety of traditional approaches. Read through them all first, then try the one that appeals to you most and see how it feels. If you like it, stick to it. Otherwise, try something else until you find one that agrees with you. Once you become comfortable with one, continue using it. After all, it's better to dig deep into one well to get water, than it is to dig several shallow wells that won't bring up anything but dirt!

> *"Mantra transforms the thinking process."*
> MUKUNDA TOM STYLES

Ajapa Japa

The simplest form of meditation is to watch and listen to the soft whooshing sound of the breath. On your inhalation, you can hear a soft "so" sound. The exhalation produces a "ham" sound. This is the Universal Mantra, also know as hansa, so hum, or so ham. So Ham is translated as meaning "I am that," and can also be chanted outloud in the following manner: "I am that, I am that, I am that, I am."

Begin to breathe deeply and slowly using the simple three-part breath (page 162) and have all your awareness on the sound your breath is repeating. After awhile, the breath will naturally slow down, and when it does, continue to follow it. After some practice, you might notice an almost imperceptable humming sound, which is part of the cosmic vibration. If you are able to hear it, move your awareness away from the breath, and focus on that beautiful hum. Tune into the cosmos to experience a bliss that will radiate peaceful vibrations out to the whole universe. Keep in mind that you are not doing this for selfish reasons, but for the peace of the entire world. Allow yourself to remain in this elevated state and feel that you are one with the Cosmic Consciousness.

Mantra Japa

The name of this meditation says a lot. *Japa* means to repeat, and a *mantra* is a sound structure, or according to Swami Sivananda, a mass of radiant energy.

Thus, mantra japa is the practice of repeating a mantra using one or more sylla-bles that represent a particular aspect of the divine vibration. The Transcendental Meditation movement, founded by Maharishi Mahesh Yogi, the Beatles' Guru, uses this technique. Repetition of a mantra is perhaps the most well known of all meditation practices. It has its basis in the understanding that sound is the medium of creation, the dynamic force of the Absolute, and as it says in the Bible, "In the beginning was the Word, and the Word was with God, and the Word was God" (*John 1:1-6*).

I like to add to that: "and the Word was mm-mmmmmm." By repeating the mantra, the mind gets focused on that one thing, instead of those 600 thoughts a minute. The most powerful mantra is "om," the cosmic hum of the universe. You can repeat "om" by itself, or add "Hari," which is another name for the Absolute. "Hari om" can be chanted out loud at first to get you started. Add a little melody to enchant the mind. Then, repeat "Hari om" silently, with just the lips moving. Gradually, let the lips become still and continue to listen internally to this simple but powerful mantra.

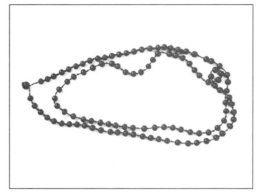

Mala beads

Another favorite mantra is "om shanthi." *Shanthi* is the Sanskrit word for peace, and not only does it mean peace, but it embodies peace. When we chant shanthi, we immediately feel the calming effect.

Once you have selected a mantra, it helps to use prayer beads to keep the mind focused. Both Western-style rosaries and Eastern-style mala beads have 108 beads (or multiples of 9 beads) with a *mehru*, or head bead. Mala comes from Sanskrit and means garland. Holding the mala in the right hand, and using the thumb and middle finger to turn the bead clockwise, repeat your mantra as you touch each successive bead. When you arrive back at the mehru, you can turn the mala around and begin again, for as long as time allows.

Mindfulness Meditation

Mindfulness meditation, which comes from the Buddhist tradition, is less about focusing on one particular thought or idea, and more about experiencing every-thing going on in consciousness. Instead of pushing away thoughts, emotions, or sensations, we open ourselves up to them—not through analysis, but through observation. When we become mindful, paying close attention to the present mo-ment, we begin to see that the mind is full of nattering and judgements. We then observe these thoughts without self-criticism and we begin to make friends with

SAMPLE FORMAT
FOR MEDITATION PRACTICE

To begin your meditation, chant "om" three times, feeling the humming vibration moving up through the top of your head. Then, recite a short prayer to center yourself. Use something from your own tradition, such as the Lord's Prayer. Or, use one the following prayers taken from ancient scripture:

Salutations to the Guru, who is auspiciousness.
Who is the embodiment of Truth, Knowledge,
  Bliss.
Who is free from world consciousness, and
  peaceful.
Who needs no support, and is Self-effulgent
  like the sun.

You are my mother and my father,
You are my brother and my friend,
You are my knowledge and my wealth,
You are my life. My light of lights you are.

Take a few slow, deep breaths, followed by three rounds of the bellows breath, with or without retention (page 172). Next, perform the nerve purifying breath (page 168) for several rounds, before embarking on ten to twenty minutes of silent meditation, choosing any technique you like.

Following the meditation, take a few slow, deep breaths once again. Finish up with a prayer of your own choosing for the peace of the world, or use the following beautiful prayers taken from the ancient Sanskrit:

May auspiciousness be unto all
May peace be unto all
May fullness be unto all
May prosperity be unto all

May happiness be unto all
May perfect health be unto all
May all see good in everyone
May all be free from suffering

Lead us from Unreal to Real
Lead us from Darkness to Light
Lead us from our fear of Death
To knowledge of Immortality.

May the entire Creation be filled with peace
  and joy, love and light.

Om Shaanthi, Shaanthi, Shaanthi

It is traditional to bow at the end of your meditation, bending the head forward toward the earth. Although its obvious benefit is to promote humility, a forward bow also has positive physiological benefits.

---

*All of these are traditional chants that go back thousands of years. The translations provided are from Swami Satchidananda's Integral Yoga Institutes, which has generously allowed me to use them here.

the mind, so that the thoughts that arise can be easily released into the nothingness from whence they came. As we detach from our thoughts, judgements, attatchments, and aversions, a feeling of joy emerges, not brought about by anything external, but by the nature of Self.

In this way, we begin to uncover Reality, or God. We see that our thoughts, feelings, and daydreams have no essential reality, no substance. Zen meditation instructor, Charlotte Jako Beck, stated "As Zen students you have a job to do, a very important job: to bring your life out of dreamland and into the real and immense reality that it is." And the great thing about mindfullness meditation is that it can be done throughout the day, in any ordinary activity—making the bed, washing the car, or taking a walk—as well as during a formal sitting meditation.

Tratak

Although tratak is actually a *kriya*, or cleansing practice, I've included it here because it's an easy meditation for beginners. Place a lighted candle at eye level, a comfortable distance in front of you as you sit for meditation. Gaze at the steady flame without straining. Keep the eyes open as long as possible, without blinking, until tears begin to flow. Then, close the eyes and continue to see the flame in your mind's eye. As soon as it fades away, re-open the eyes and again begin to gaze at the steady flame. Continue in this way for a while, then let the eyes close and naturally go into a deep meditation.

This type of meditation on a form—the candle—can also be done using a picture of a beloved saint or teacher, a sacred symbol, such as a cross or Jewish star, or a *yantra*, which is a mystic symbol in the form of a geometric diagram of the cosmos, revealed to the mystics in deep meditation. Use the same technique as gazing at the flame, opening and closing the eyes gently while maintaining concentration on the image. Tratak is a very effective method for controlling the mind and developing will power, and it has the added benefit of improving the eyesight.

Erich Schiffman, contemporary Yoga teacher and author of *Moving into Stillness*, encourages the technique of tratak using a mirror, making the object of concentration your own image! Place the mirror at eye level and gaze into your own eyes. You might be surprised by what you see there!

Likit Japa

If you're feeling a little restless, you might enjoy the practice of likit japa. Using a pen and paper, perhaps in a special notebook used just for this purpose, begin to write a mantra you enjoy, such as God is love, Alleluia, or So Ham. Rewrite the mantra again and again on the paper. Then begin chanting it, either silently or softly, while writing. Distractions are minimized as the mind, tongue, hands, and eyes are all engaged with the mantra. Be neat and regular in your letters, and have a uniform style of writing. Or, if you are feeling really creative, you can use the mantra in a design, or even draw a picture with the mantras. Personally, I call this technique sacred doodling. When I'm stuck on hold with the phone company or someone else, I find it a useful way to keep my peace, which you probably know is not always the easiest thing to do!

> *"When you walk, let your feet kiss the ground."*
> THICH NHAT HANH

Walking Meditation

During the ten-day silent retreats at Yogaville, there are three meditation sessions a day. At the noon meditation, many retreatants opt for the walking meditation. Participants walk slowly, silently, and intentionally in single file, while silently repeating a chosen mantra. Usually the eyelids are almost closed, aiding in keeping the awareness within. The breath is slow and steady. The footsteps are loosely synchronized, which creates a feeling that truly we all are one. This practice helps to bring the experience of mantra japa (page 188) into our everyday life. You can also try this technique on your own if you can find a quiet place where you won't be disturbed by intrusions, such as people bumping into you on the street, or traffic endangering your life!

Another approach to walking meditation is to keep the eyes open, trying to take in and experience everything in your path. Pay attention to the exquisite details of the life around you. This has the effect of heightening the senses to a spiritual level, allowing a radiant joy to emerge.

Laughing Meditation

Cortisol is a stress hormone, and it can be toxic to the heart muscle. Laughter has been proven to reduce cortisol in the bloodstream, inducing a relaxing effect on the entire body. Laughing meditation is done in a group, with everyone lying head-to-head on the floor, bodies stretching out like spokes of a large wheel. The leader might begin with a few jokes until the group has warmed up, feels uninhibited, and is laughing for no reason. He or she then continues gently pulling the group along the laughter track, with members of the group instigating laughter on their own in guffaws, giggles, hoots, hollers, or shrieks. You'll want to laugh when you hear the incredible varieties of laughter! My friend Saraswati attended a session recently and said, "My whole body was tingling at the end of laughing meditation! My arms were tingling, my legs were tingling, even the tip of my nose was tingling!" This type of group meditation typically goes on for about thirty minutes, and then might end with a few minutes of blissful silence and perhaps a few closing chants.

Yoga Nidra Meditation

Yoga Nidra is a form of guided meditation that leads to the awareness of subtler levels of mind and body as accumulated tensions are released and spontaneous healing occurs. Also known as the Yogic Sleep, Yoga Nidra is an extended deep relaxation that can be practiced for as long as time permits. It generally begins with the student relaxing in the supine corpse (page 62), as the teacher instructs him or her to tense and relax all the different parts of the body, one after the other. Following that, the student is told to mentally assess the body and release any hidden tensions, deepening the feeling of relaxation. This process of going deeper into stillness allows the body to "right" itself. It can also allow for emotional healing. I always try to include Yoga Nidra in all my classes—I like to think of it as the dessert of the class.

Kirtan

Kirtan is chanting a mantra with feeling. It can be done alone or in a group, with a large band or just some simple finger cymbals. Kirtan is one of my favorite practices, and when leading a chanting session at the ashram, I encourage everyone to chant with their whole heart! It's not about how pretty your voice is, or whether you're singing in tune. Whatever you put into your chanting, you will receive back tenfold in joy and ecstasy.

Krishna Das, Jai Uttal, Deva Premal, Wah!, and Bhagavan Das are all excellent kirtanists who have brought the joys of Indian-style chanting to the Western seeker, creating an inspiring East-West fusion. Their recordings can give you a taste of this joyful practice, but to really get the full effect, chant with others. The group energy creates a huge spiritual current, and helps to purify the heart and elevate the mind. It is one of the major practices of Bhakti Yoga, which is discussed in greater detail beginning on page 199.

Deep Relaxation (*Yoga Nidra*) Script

Lying on your back in the supine corpse, allow your body to sink into the floor—into mother earth. You're letting go of all tension, with no holding anywhere. Feel that the floor is doing all the work to support you completely. The legs are wide, with the arms alongside the body, a few inches away from the sides. Have the palms facing up. If the palms have a tendency to roll in and down, open the shoulders by squeezing the bottom of the shoulder blades together under the body.

In this guided relaxation, Yoga Nidra, we're going to tense and relax every part of the body. Imagine yourself squeezing out residual toxins in the system. Then, we'll go over the body once more, this time at the mental level. We won't actually move a single muscle. And though you'll be resting deeply, try not to fall asleep.

To begin, bring all your awareness to your right leg. Begin to stretch it out, making it long. Then tense it up. Point the toes. Raise the leg an inch or two off the floor and make it tight. Longer . . . tighter . . . and release. Let the leg plop to the floor, as if it were a branch cut from a tree. Roll it gently from side to side, and then forget the right leg. Bring the awareness to the left leg. Stretch it out. Raise it up a few inches off the floor. Point the toes. Tense every muscle in the leg . . . a little tighter . . . a little longer . . . and release. Drop the leg back to the floor, roll it from side to side, and then forget the legs.

Begin to think about your right arm. Stretch it out. Stretch out the fingers of the right hand. Tighten the whole arm and lift it

a few inches off the ground. Make a fist and squeeze it tight. Make the arm longer . . . tighter . . . and release. Roll it gently from side to side, and then forget about it. Bring the awareness to the left arm. Stretch it out. Stretch out the fingers. Tense up the whole arm. Make a fist with the left hand and lift the arm up off the floor. Make it longer . . . tighter . . . and release. Let it roll softly from side to side, and then forget about the arms.

Move the awareness to the buttocks. Tense the muscles tight . . . squeezing tighter . . . almost as if you're about to rise right up off the floor. Squeeze tighter . . . and release.

Think about your belly. Inhale into the abdomen. Fill the belly with as much air as you can bring in. Fill it up like a big balloon. Let it stick way out. Hold the breath there . . . then open the mouth and let it all gush out. Release.

Now focus the attention on the upper chest. Fill it with as much air as you can bring in . . . a little bit more . . . hold it . . . hold it. And release.

Leave your arms in place, but begin to roll the shoulders forward, bringing them together under your chin. Squeeze the shoulders . . . and release.

Shift your awareness to the face. Open the mouth. Stick out the tongue. Raise the eyebrows. Stretch out all the muscles of the face . . . and release. Now make a prune face. Squeeze the muscles of the face tight . . . tighter . . . and release. Gently roll the head from side to side a couple of times to make sure there aren't any kinks in the neck. Then bring the head to center.

Have a check on the body and make any minor adjustments you'd like to before we go into our mental scan. From this point on, we're not going to move anything at the physical level. We'll deepen our relaxation by bringing our awareness to every part of the body. If there are any residual tensions, we'll let go mentally.

So, begin by checking the soles of the feet. If you find any tension, let it melt away. Check the toes. Are there any rebellious muscles that are still holding on to tension? If so, gently suggest a release. Relax the tops of the feet, the arches, and the heels. Relax the ankles. . . .

Moving up the leg, relax the shins, the calves, the knees, and the backs of the knees. Relax the thighs. Then, forget the legs and move the awareness to the palms of the hands. Check for any tension and mentally let it go. Relax the forearms, elbows, and upper arms.

Forget the arms and bring the awareness to the buttocks, hips, and groin. Release any little tensions there. Relax the belly, ribcage, and upper chest. Think about the muscles that support the spine, and let them soften and relax deeply. Release any tension in the back ribs, shoulder blades, and shoulders.

Soften and relax the neck. Relax all the parts of the head including the chin, the jaw, the ears, the temples, and the cheeks. Relax the lips, the tongue, the nose, and the eyes.

Relax the eyebrows and the space between the eyebrows. Relax the forehead and the crown of the head.

Take a minute or two to really relish the feeling of ease and comfort in the body.

Then, bring the awareness to the breath. Take a couple of minutes to feel its gentle flow in and out of the body, without trying to control it in any way.

Now, slowly shift your awareness to the thoughts in the mind. Begin to watch whatever comes up, without any judgment. . . . Become the silent witness of the mind. . . . This is the part of you that is always happy and peaceful. It is your true nature. It is awareness itself, beyond the mind and body. Rest now, and be that peace. (Pause for four or five minutes.)

Om. Begin to bring the mind back. . . . As the mind becomes more active, it will wake up the breath. . . . Let the breath deepen. As you do, the body will want to wake up, as well. Begin to wake the body by wiggling the toes and fingers. Stretch out a little. Maybe have a little yawn.

When you feel ready, begin to roll over to one side, and at your own pace, gradually come back to a seated position. Keep your eyes closed for another minute or two as you observe the peaceful feeling created by your Yoga Nidra practice. If you have more time, do some pranayama breathing practices before going back into your day.

Self-Inquiry Meditation

This is a meditation on *you*. Sitting comfortably in a relaxed position, begin to question yourself. Ask, "Who am I?" Hmm—that's a tough one! "If I'm not my thoughts, who am I?" "If I'm not my job, who am I?" Continue to negate all you call "mine," and try to stand apart from these thoughts of identification. The ancient Yogis used a technique called *Neti-Neti*, meaning not this, not this. "Do I define myself by my position in the family? Not this, not this. Am I this body I live in? Not this, not this." This aloofness is a kind of Nirvana, or liberation, and is the path of Jnana Yoga—the Yoga of wisdom. It is a simple practice perhaps, but it is deeply profound. It can be briefly summed up in a short chant I learned at the feet of my Guru:

> *I'm not the body; I'm not the mind,*
> *Immortal Self I am.*
> *In all conditions, I am Knowledge,*
> *Bliss Absolute.*

As we continue to cut cords and detach from forms such as the body, the possessions, and the mind, we begin to see that some part of us is observing the process. We are the field of consciousness that gives rise to the content. According to the Yoga philosophers, that awareness is the same awareness that we call God, or Supreme Consciousness.

Ramana Maharshi, one of the most famous sages of the twentieth century, gave advice on Jnana *sadhana,* or practice, by saying, "What is essential in any sadhana practice is to try to bring back the running mind and fix it on one thing only. Why, then, should it not be brought back and fixed in self-attention? That alone is Self-Inquiry. That is all that is to be done."

Well, that's a bit of a relief! I can grok that. I admit I'm not a philosopher. I'm a true-to-form Virgo and I like practical things that can be filed and organized. (As my friend Al jokingly says, "There's room for you at the bottom!") That's why my favorite Yoga text is Patanjali's ancient *Yoga Sutras.* It boils down all these meditation techniques into the one, important, recurring theme: When we quiet the thought-waves in the mind, we abide in our own true nature, which is that same Cosmic Consciousness as God. And being a songwriter, I appreciate the pithyness of the sutras. In matters of philosophy, the less that is said, the better.

THE CULMINATION OF MEDITATION

In the *Yoga Sutras,* Patanjali states that the culmination of meditation is *samadhi,* or self-realization. This eighth limb on the tree of Yoga is an indescribable experience in which the meditator, which Patanjali refers to as "the knower," merges with the knowable and with knowledge itself. All the different meditation techniques decribed in this chapter are presented to offer you options. There isn't any one "right" way on this path toward happiness and enlightenment. As Sri Swami Satchidananda said, use "anything that delights the mind."

For now, you may want to stick to your Hatha practice exclusively. As you gain in confidence, however, you may become curious about practicing sense withdrawal, concentration, and meditation. Go at your own pace and enjoy the journey.

Chapter 8

Service and Devotion

What makes *Big Yoga* "big" is more than its physical adaptations for bigger bodies. *Big Yoga* is also "big," because it is expansive and includes a variety of practices along the Yoga spectrum. We have now investigated several Yoga practices, including Hatha Yoga, which includes the Yoga postures; Raja Yoga, which teaches us the practices of the eight-limbed tree of Yoga and its ultimate goal of controlling the mind and senses; and Jnana Yoga, which is the study of the self. The next two valuable areas of study are Karma

> *"Love is the best offering that a human being can make, and all material objects are simply a token of one's love and faith."*
> PANDIT RAJMANI TIGUNAIT

Yoga (service) and Bhakti Yoga (devotion). We can't all be great Hatha Yogis, and not everyone is suited for the disciplines of Raja and Jnana Yoga. However, everyone can love and serve their fellow human beings, and for those with an emotional nature, the practices of Bhakti and Karma Yoga might be a good fit.

KARMA YOGA—THE YOGA OF SERVICE

The simple practice of Karma Yoga is based on giving without any expectation of receiving. John Lennon sang, "Instant Karma's gonna get you!" And since then, the word "Karma" has seemingly become part of everyone's vocabulary. It comes from the Sanskrit root word *kri*, meaning "to act." Thus, any physical or mental action, as well as the result of that action, is Karma. It is an immutable law of nature. It is cause and effect, and it is all intertwined. We experience the fruits of our past actions, while simultaneously creating new Karma. There is also Karma lying in wait—the sum total of past actions, good and bad, which will present itself when the time is right for its expression.

LEARN TO THINK LIKE A KARMA YOGI

We usually think of Karma as the visible, tangible results of our actions. They are Karma, but there is more to it than that. All of our actions also carry invisible after-effects, because they leave impressions in our minds. This is why aphorisms such as "Love thy neighbor as thyself," and "Do unto others as you would have them do unto you," have become universal. By cultivating good thoughts and good deeds, no matter how seemingly insignificant, we affect the whole world, directly or indirectly.

Karma Yogis seek to renounce the fruits of their actions and offer all the results of their efforts to God or humanity. They do things simply for the sake and joy of doing them. Every action becomes a sacrifice and an offering. Non-attachment (*vairagya*)—not to be confused with indifference—is the key to practicing Karma Yoga. It is an attitude of not clinging to things or ideas—of non-possessiveness. This fosters humility, diminishes the ego, and keeps you in the present moment.

Karma Yoga's practice of selfless service relieves you of the burden of judging the results of your actions. You can take the mental attitude that God (Higher Power, Universal Intelligence . . . take your pick of expression) is making you do everything, so if the results are good, it's because God made them good. And if the results are bad, God probably had a reason for things to turn out that way.

BEGIN YOUR KARMA YOGA PRACTICE

To get a taste for Karma Yoga, Swami Satchidananda offered this challenge: Try to make a commitment to have a whole day of selfless service every so often. When you get up, begin your day with a prayer that every effort you make you will offer to God or the greater good. Meditate on what you're doing, and watch your feelings and your thoughts. When you take your shower, think, "I am washing the temple of the living God." When you eat your breakfast, think, "I am feeding myself a healthy breakfast so I'll be fit for a good day's work." Make work your worship.

When you practice Karma Yoga, you will quickly learn your weaknesses, because while serving others, some of your negative tendencies and bad habits may come to light. For instance, when doing the morning meal's dishes, do you find yourself complaining that your significant other forgot to bring his or her bowl to the sink? Are you cross when scrubbing the oatmeal that's stuck to the pan? Do you look for someone to blame when you realize you've run out of dish soap? These are all ways the ego pulls us out of the present moment. But this can actually be a good thing! Once you recognize that you have allowed the mind to move out of non-judgment and into negativity, you can work to correct this tendency. In an example from my own life, I was unaware of my habit to be overly loud until I met my husband, who was basically a quiet type. My noisiness began to annoy him, and so he called me on it. I then began to pay better attention and bring awareness to the quality of my voice in order to create more harmony in our home. My guru called this "rubbing and scrubbing," and it is something all Karma Yogis experience.

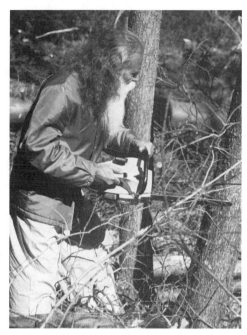

Swami Satchidananda with a chain saw

The practice of Karma Yoga cultivates equanimity and helps us become steady, so that we're not blown about by the winds of change: profit and loss, good and evil, praise and blame, heat and cold, pleasure and pain. It allows the innate joy of our being to come to the surface of our consciousness, and raises everyday activities to a higher dimension through contemplative awareness. Then, what used to be the "ordinary" acts of making a sandwich, washing the dishes, driving the car, paying the bills, or taking out the trash, become forms of contemplation and worship.

Mahatma Gandhi was an exemplary Karma Yogi. He served India tirelessly, embracing his destiny without rancor. He suffered tremendously during long, austere fasts in order to influence Britain to give India its independence. He read the Bhagavad-Gita daily and felt no distain for any labor, embracing equally the duties of Prime Minister and the humble weaver. Mother Teresa is another example of a modern day Karma Yogi. When we model our behaviors after inspiring people such as these, we can begin to take on some of their qualities and begin to bring our Yoga off the mat and into our lives.

BHAKTI YOGA—THE YOGA OF DEVOTION

Bhakti means devotion, and just as Karma Yoga is action for action's sake, Bhakti Yoga is love for love's sake. In the practices of Bhakti Yoga, the devotee attaches himself to his *Ishta-Devata*—chosen form of the Divine—through song or celebratory worship, and develops a supreme, sacred love. The basic principle of Bhakti is that, in the words of Buddha, "As we think, so we become." So, for example, if a Christian sings the praises of Jesus unceasingly, he or she will begin to embody the qualities of sacrifice, love, and compassion that we associate with Jesus. Combined, the practices of Karma Yoga and Bhakti Yoga help to purify the mind of the Yogi, making him or her fit for the more advanced practices of Jnana and Raja Yoga.

Bhakti Songs of Praise

Bhakti songs of praise open the heart and help to destroy spiritual impurities such as greed, anger, hate, jealousy, depression, and other negative emotions. They are common to many religious traditions, including Christianity, Judaism, and more. And who hasn't felt uplifted by the singing of a carol at Christmas time, the National Anthem at a sporting event, or Dayenu at a Passover Seder?

"The thought manifests as the word,
The word manifests as the deed,
The deed develops into habit,
And habit hardens in character,
So watch the thought and its ways with care,
And let it spring from love,
Born out of concern for all beings . . .
As the shadow follows the body,
As we think, so we become."
BUDDHA (FROM THE *DHAMMAPADA*)

One of the main practices in Bhakti Yoga is a kind of repetitive singing known as chanting. You may have been made aware of chanting by the Hare Krishnas, who bring chanting into the streets with their orange robes, bare feet, and jingling cymbals, singing the ancient chant "Hare Krishna, Hare Krishna, Krishna Krishna, Hare Hare." Interestingly, the Eastern practice of kirtan—a type of call and response chanting—is undergoing a fusion with Western music, and is becoming a popular music genre! This is helping those of us who are living and working in the world to stay in frequent contact with the Divine Names of God, such as Krishna, Buddha, Jesus, Mother Mary, and thousands of other Holy names.

I notice after even a short time of chanting or singing, I continue to hear the mantras and chants in my mind, sometimes for days. This helps to recharge my spiritual battery. Chanting is especially helpful during times of distress, especially conflict with loved ones. When the mind is on fire with anger, looping on a negative thought, kirtan can be a wonderful tonic. It is also helpful to alleviate the symptoms of depression. Chanting done with devotion is one way of worshipping the Divine. It opens the heart, calms the mind, enlivens the senses, and creates a feeling of inner happiness.

Common Thread Among Various Religions

All religions have a Bhakti element. Mass, or Holy Communion, as celebrated by Roman Catholics and other Christian churches is a good example. In its celebration, our senses are engaged in worship through the lighting of incense and candles, the offering of prayers, the taking of the bread and wine, and the beautiful flowers at the altar. Hindus also have a special ceremony called *Puja*, which, surprisingly, has many of the same elements as Mass: flower petals, prayers of glory and devotion, candles or a special *ghee* lamp, incense, and special food called *Prasad*. Moreover, I was surprised and delighted when I attended my first Passover Seder to realize that many of these same elements of worship found their place there, as well: blessed food and wine, light, prayers and songs of glory, and gratitude for the grace of God.

The list of religions that share in these Bhakti elements goes on and on. Muslims offer themselves to God several times a day as they bow down in humility and reverence. Sufis are famous for their ecstatic dancing during worship. Buddhists show their devotion by chanting, bowing at images of the Buddha, offering flowers and chants, and taking pilgrimages to sites made holy by Buddha's birth, enlightenment, and death. And in the Far East, Daoists have holy diagrams and recite and chant sacred texts, both historical and ethical.

Some schools of thought claim that Bhakti Yoga should be given prominence over meditation. In the Hare Krishna movement, for example, chanting is the main spiritual practice. Regardless of its differing priority levels, though, the path

> *"Truth is One,*
> *Paths Are Many."*
> SRI SWAMI SATCHIDANANDA

of devotion is widely known as the easiest way to emancipation, especially in the modern times. Instead of total identification with God, as in Jnana Yoga, Bhaktas prefer to look upon the Divine as separate, so they can continue the play of worship. I think it's a little bit like playing with paper dolls, where you act the part of mother. You dress your doll, play with her, speak for her, and have a dialog with her, as if she is separate from you. That's *lila*, the play. In life, we are all playing a role in which we pretend to be separate and independent from God, but, according to Yoga philosophy, we are all One. If we know we are all One, it gets a little boring, so we take on our personalities and habits and pretend we are different from God, so we can have a little fun.

TRY IT. YOU MIGHT LIKE IT!

Bhakti and Karma Yoga go hand in hand. If you live in an area where there are Yoga studios (and who doesn't?), find out when they do their chanting and go experience its intoxicating effect! You will enjoy the music and meet some nice people. You might also consider volunteering at your Yoga center for some service. Offer yourself. Get connected with other people who are seeking self-knowledge. Become part of The Happening!

Big Yoga offers you all these options, from the physical to the mystical. I recommend you try a little of everything, and approach your own personal evolution on many fronts. Do a little chanting, a little asana practice, a little self-less service, and a little meditation. Find the practices that you relish and go for it!

Conclusion

We all want to be happy, but unless we are truly healthy, how can we enjoy life? When the body is achy, stiff, and susceptible to frequent bouts of colds and flus, life can be pretty miserable. Beginning a simple, profound practice of Yoga can literally turn your life around. With regular Yoga practice, you will begin to thrive. You'll regain confidence in yourself and aquire a *jois de vivre* akin to how you felt as a child, without any worries or troubles.

We have become a nation of consumers—hoping the new Lexus vehicle, Prada bag, or Rolex watch will bring us happiness. For awhile, these material indulgences do work. But ultimately, the joyous feelings they give us fade and we are driven to find something new to fill that void. Thus, this quest for momentary pleasure becomes constant and never fully satisfying. My advice to you is to stop looking externally. There is already a permanent joy inside all of us!

Yoga can uncover this lasting happiness by healing us physically, emotionally, and mentally. My friend and author, Dr. Sandra McClanahan, says, "Happiness is in the happening!" And author Eckhart Tolle talks about "the power of now" in his book of the same name. When we are in the "now," we are free of the bondage of our judgments, our considerations, and our disappointments, which all create veils of darkness covering our inner light. Similarly, Sri Swami Satchidananda spoke of the "golden present," saying that only in the present moment can we find the "peace that passes all understanding." Yoga practice brings the Yogi into the knowledge of the Self in communion with the Divine. Since this Cosmic Consciousness, or God, is infinite, it can only be experienced when the individual rises above his or her limited personality, which is possible when the tools of Yoga are used with practice and compassion.

I have seen Yoga work healing miracles with my students. One of my favorite students is a sixty-seven-year-old plus-size woman who had stopped exercising at age sixty. When she first came to my class, she had trouble getting up and down off the floor, her mind was full of chatter, and her knee was painful and unstable. In addition, she had a variety of little aches and pains and some trouble sleeping. Determined to improve, she began regularly attending class and experimenting with props, chairs, blankets, pillows, and wedges. Her body responded beautifully, becoming more supple and graceful with every session. Her mind became calm and focused, and her will became unshakeable. Today, she is a certified *Big Yoga* instructor with students of her own, and she is spreading the message of Yoga to others like her in need of healing.

By reading this book, you have taken the first step toward becoming a healthier, happier person. You have looked at the pictures of the poses and have even read the chapter on meditation! Now, however, you must actually *do* Yoga. And not just once, but frequently. So what are you waiting for? Start now! And as you embark on this journey toward liberation, I wish for you the joy of inhabiting a healthy body, the grace of a teacher to guide you, and the eternal happiness that is your true nature. Om shaanthi, shaanthi, shaanthi.

Om and Prem,

Meeraji

P.O. Box 237
Glenn, Michigan 49416
Website: www.bigyogaonline.com

> *"Health, not disease, is your birthright;*
> *Strength, not weakness is your heritage,*
> *courage not sorrow; peace not restlessness;*
> *knowledge not ignorance.*
> *May you attain this birthright,*
> *this divine heritage,*
> *to shine as fully developed Yogis,*
> *radiating joy, peace and knowledge everywhere."*
> SRI SWAMI SATCHIDANANDA

Basic Yoga Glossary

acharya. Spiritual teacher.

ahimsa. Non-injury; non-harming.

akasha. Space; ether.

ananda. Bliss; ecstasy.

asana. A comfortable, steady posture that promotes a feeling of stillness within.

ashram. A Hindu term for religious retreats where students are guided by spiritually qualified, ordained swamis.

Ashtanga Yoga. The eight-fold path of Yoga as described in Patanjali's Yoga Sutras, including: yama, niyama, asana, pranayama, pratyhara, dharana, dhyana, and samadhi.

atman. The soul, or self.

Ayurveda. Ancient Indian system of traditional medicine that uses herbs, diet, massage, and Yoga to keep the body in balance.

bandha. Lock; the contracting of muscles and organs to build up energy internally.

Bhakti Yoga. The Yoga of devotion and love.

Brahman. Supreme consciousness; absolute truth or reality.

chakra. Circles or wheels of energy in the body.

dharma. The path of righteousness; your spiritual duty.

diksha. Initiation given to a student by a master or guru.

dosha. Three basic constitutions of the body, according to Ayurvedic theory: kapha, pitta, and vata.

guru. Remover of darkness; one who is spiritually enlightened and able to help devotees uncover their own inner light.

Hatha. Sun and moon, heat and coolness; usually refers to the practices of Hatha Yoga: asanas, pranayama, mudra, bandha, and kriya.

japa. Continuous chanting or recitation of a mantra or prayer.

jnana. Wisdom; knowledge.

kapha. One of the three basic constitutions of the body, according to Ayurvedic theory; related to earth, water, and bodily fluids.

karma. Actions and the fruits of actions.

kirtan. The practice of chanting the names of God.

koshas. The coverings or sheaths of the physical and astral bodies.

kriyas. Yogic cleansing practices.

kundalini. Latent energy stored at the base of the spine—said to be coiled like a snake—that is released upward as a result of Yoga practice, resulting in feelings of joy and peace.

mantra. A sound structure that settles the mind; incantation.

moksha. Liberation from the cycles of birth and death.

moola. Root; refers to the first chakra at the area of the perineum where kundalini is stored.

mudra. Seal; postures used to seal energy in the body.

nadi. Subtle energy channels throughout the body, similar to the meridians in acupuncture.

nirvana. A state of liberation from the ego-self; a state of awareness beyond time and space.

niyama. The second limb of Patanjali's eight-limbed Yoga tree. It encompasses five Yogic observances or disciplines, including purity, contentment, austerity, study, and devotion.

Om. The name of the sound of the subtle vibration of the universe, from which all matter is created; the chief mantra.

ojas. Vigor; the subtle energy that builds from Yoga practice.

pitta. One of the doshas according to Ayurvedic theory; prominent characteristic is fire; governs transformation.

pranayama. Breathing techniques used to restrain (yama) vital energy (prana).

pratyahara. The fifth-limb on Pantajali's Yoga tree; the discipline of withdrawing the mind from the senses.

Raja Yoga. The royal path of Yoga, as outlined in Patanjali's *Yoga Sutras*; practices leading to mastery of the mind and senses.

samadhi. The ultimate goal of Yoga, in which concentration merges with the object of concentration; a complete absorption in God or Supreme Consciousness.

samskara. Impressions, which come to consciousness due to the senses, that are left in the mind and are the basis for our habits and beliefs; memory or restlessness of the mind.

sankalpa. Firm decision; vow.

sanyasi. A monk or swami; one who renounces the world and takes initiation into the Holy Order of Sannyas.

santosha. Contentment.

sat. Truth.

satchidananda. Truth (sat), knowledge (chid), and bliss (ananda); the nature of the Ultimate.

satsang. A gathering of seekers of Truth, usually with the purpose of listening to, or about, a Realized Being.

shakti. Vital force; energy.

shanthi. The peace of God "that passes all understanding."

soham. The mantra of the breath: So (the inhale) Ham (the exhale); roughly translated to mean "I am that."

sutras. Thread; refers to the nearly 200 aphorisms, known as the *Yoga Sutras*, compiled by the sage and physician, Maharishi Patanjali in the second or third century A.D.

swami. A monk, renunciate, or spiritual master.

ujjayi. The hissing breath, caused by gently closing the glottis.

vata. One of the three doshas according to the Ayurveda theory; pertains to air and movement.

Vedanta. A school of philosophy based on Vedic scripture, which believes in the Oneness of All; non-dualism.

Vedas. Four ancient texts—Rig, Yajur, Sama, and Atharva—revealed to ancient sages and saints of India, which explain every aspect of human life and the Life Divine.

yantra. A visual depiction of a mantra; mandala, or sacred design.

yama. The first limb Patanjali's Yoga tree. It encompasses a set of five Yogic abstinences, including non-violence, truthfulness, non-stealing, chastity, and non-greed.

Yoga. From the Sanskrit, meaning to yoke or join together; uniting body, mind, and spirit.

Yoga Nidra. Restorative deep relaxation in which the body and mind are at rest, but not asleep in the normal sense.

Resources

This book has a wide range of information on Yoga and meditation , but if you would like to learn more about these subjects, or find out more about how Yoga can have a positive effect on your health, this resource section is for you. In it you will find recommended reading materials, DVDs, CDs, websites, ashrams and retreat centers, and places to buy plus-size activewear. And this is only a small sample of what is available in bookstores, online, and at your local library. Enjoy the feast!

RECOMMENDED READING

If you would like to further explore any of the subjects covered in *Big Yoga,* I recommend reading the following books. The books listed range from classical philosophical Yoga texts, to books specifically about Hatha Yoga, to books about how to use Yoga as a wellness tool. Some of these resources have been my friends for many years, and now have notes scribbled in the margins and pages folded over or bookmarked. Others are newer to me, but are a welcome addition to my library. Almost all of the following titles can be found and purchased on Amazon.com.

Asana Pranayama Mudra Bandha by Swami Satyananda Saraswati

Autobiography of a Yogi by Paramahansa Yogananda

Beyond Words by Sri Swami Satchidananda

The Complete Illustrated Book of Yoga by Swami Vishnu-Devananda

Dr. Yoga: A Complete Guide to the Medical Benefits of Yoga by Nirmala Heriza, C. Noel Bairey Merz, and Dean Ornish M.D.

Eat More, Weigh Less: Dr. Dean Ornish's Life Choice Program for Losing Weight Safely While Eating Abundantly by Dean Ornish M.D.

The Golden Present: Daily Inspirational Readings by Sri Swami Satchidananda

The Healing Path of Yoga: Time-Honored Wisdom and Scientifically Proven Methods That Alleviate Stress, Open Your Heart, and Enrich Your Life by Nischala Joy Devi, Dean Ornish M.D., and Shaye Areheart

Inside the Yoga Sutras: A Comprehensive Sourcebook for the Study and Practice of Patanjali's Yoga Sutras by Reverend Jaganath Carrera

Integral Yoga Hatha by Sri Swami Satchidananda

Kiss Guide to Yoga by Shakta Kaur Khalsa

The Living Gita: The Complete Bhagavad Gita—A Commentary for Modern Readers by Sri Swami Satchidananda

Living Yoga by Georg Fuerstein

Mega Yoga by Megan Garcia

Relax and Renew: Restful Yoga for Stressful Times by Judith Lasater

The Secret Power of Yoga: A Woman's Guide to the Heart and Spirit of the Yoga Sutras by Nischala Joy Devi

Stress Diet and Your Heart: A Lifetime Program for Healing Your Heart without Drugs or Surgery by Dean Ornish M.D.

Structural Yoga Therapy: Adapting to the Individual by Mukunda Stiles

Surgery and Its Alternatives: How to Make the Right Choices for Your Health by Sandra and David McLanahan

Yoga as Medicine: The Yogic Prescription for Health and Healing by Yoga Journal and Timothy McCall M.D.

The Yoga Sutras of Patanjali: Commentary on the Raja Yoga Sutras by Sri Swami Satchidananda

Yoga Sutras of Patanjali: With Great Respect and Love by Mukunda Stiles

Yoga: The Spirit and Practice of Moving into Stillness by Erich Schiffmann

DVD'S

While there are hundreds of Yoga DVDs on the market, most are challenging for the larger body. So, be sure to watch videos before trying them, to see for yourself if they're appropriate for your body. Also, in addition to the DVDs listed below, which you can find on Amazon.com, you can go to YouTube.com to see free Yoga classes online.

Big Yoga: Flex-Ability with Meera Patricia Kerr

Big Yoga Hatha One with Meera Patricia Kerr

Heavyweight Yoga with Abbey Lenz

Yoga: Just My Size with Megan Garcia

Yoga for Round Bodies with Linda Demarco and Genia Pauli Haddon

CD'S FOR CHANTING

Chanting purifies the mind and opens the heart. If you've never tried it, you may enjoy the following albums by various inspiring artists, available through Amazon.com. If you find you like it, look for a Yoga studio in your area where you can enjoy this devotional practice with others. It will light you up!

Chants of India by Ravi Shankar and George Harrison

Cool Dual Live with Shyamdas by Kirtan and Satsang with Shyamdas

Footprints by Jai Uttal

Kirtan: The Art and Practice of Ecstatic Chant by Jai Uttal

Live On Earth by Krishna Das

Love is Space by Deva Premal

The Love Window by Shantala

Meditation Series: Chanting by Wah!

Now by Bhagavan Das

One Track Heart by Krishna Das

Pilgrim Heart by Krishna Das

Siva Station by Jai Uttal

Sunset Kirtan (Volumes 1, 2, and 3) by Bhagavan Das

Thus Sang Sant Tulsidas by Sadguru Sant Keshavadas

CD'S FOR YOGA PRACTICE

When you're practicing Yoga at home, it's sometimes nice to have some music softly playing in the background. Here are a few suggestions of CDs that I like because the music is slow-paced and doesn't draw your attention to it, which helps keep focus on Yoga.

Ambient 2: The Plateaux of Mirror by Brian Eno and Harold Budd

Jai Ma: White Swan Yoga Masters Volume 2 (Feminine Voices Sing of the Divine) by Various Artists

Music for Yoga and Other Joys by Jai Uttal and Ben Leinbach

Omniscient Om by Meera Patricia Kerr

The Room by Harold Budd

WEBSITES

There are over 64 million results when you search for "Yoga" in Google. So, I thought I would help narrow down your search a bit! The following websites are some of my personal favorites.

www.abc-of-yoga.com

www.sivananda.org

www.bigyogaonline.com

www.swamisatchidananda.org

www.harekrishna.com

www.yogahealthbooks.com

www.integralyogaprograms.org

www.yogajournal.com

www.iyiva.org

www.yogaalliance.org

www.iyta.org

www.yogaville.org

www.lotus.org

ASHRAMS AND RETREAT CENTERS

When you find yourself getting more serious about Yoga, you may want to immerse yourself in the Yogic lifestyle. Spending time at an ashram or Yoga retreat can boost your skills,as well as your resolve to keep practicing. Here are some suggestions:

Amrit Yoga Institute
23855 NE County Road 314
PO Box 5340
Salt Springs, FL 32134
Tel: 352-685-3001
Website: www.amrityoga.org

Himalayan Institute
952 Bethany Turnpike
Honesdale, PA 18431
Tel: 800-822-4547
Website: www.himalayaninstitute.org

Kripalu Center for Yoga and Health
PO Box 309
Stockbridge, MA 01262
Tel: 866-200-5203
Website: www.kripalu.org

Satchidananda Ashram at Yogaville
108 Yogaville Way
Buckingham, VA 23921
Tel: 434-969-3121 ext. 108
Website: www.integralyogaprograms.
    org

Sivananda Ashram Yoga Farm
14651 Ballantree
Grass Valley, CA 95949
Tel: 530-272-9322, 800-469-9642
Website: www.sivanandayogafarm.
    org

Sivananda Ashram Yoga Retreat
P.O. Box N7550
Paradise Island
Nassau, Bahamas

Tel: 242-363-2902, 800-441-2096
Website: www.sivanandabahamas.org

PLUS-SIZE ACTIVEWEAR

It's getting easier to find fashionable, comfortable work-out clothes in larger sizes. Several places are carrying them these days, but the stores listed below will get your search off to a good start.

Always for Me: www.alwaysforme.com

Danskin: www.danskin.com

Junonia: www.junonia.com

Eddie Bauer: www.eddiebauer.com

Lands End: www.landsend.com

J.C. Penney: www.jcpenney.com

Old Navy: www.oldnavy.gap.com

YOGA PROPS

Yoga props, such as meditation benches, mats, and pillows, are available through several different outlets these days. The following website is a great place to start your search.

www.yogaaccessories.com

Index

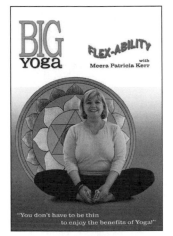
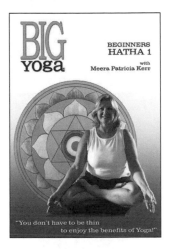
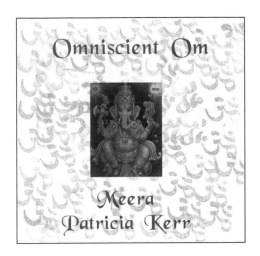

THE DŌ-IN WAY
Gentle Exercises to Liberate the Body, Mind, and Spirit
Michio Kushi

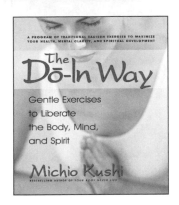

Dō-In is an ancient traditional exercise for the cultivation of physical health, mental serenity, and spirituality. Over the last 5,000 years, it has served as the origin of such well-known disciplines as shiatsu, acupuncture, moxibustion, yogic exercises, and meditation. Literally meaning to pull and stretch, Dō-In originated as a way of achieving longevity and attaining the highest potential of mental and spiritual development.

Dō-In techniques are a series of successive motions designed to harmonize body systems. *The Dō-In Way* details the fundamental aspects of this exercise, which involves breathing, posture, and self-massage and manipulation to stimulate body systems. The gentle application of pressure on the body's meridians corresponds directly with physical processes, and allows for the conditioning and stimulation of internal organs. This is a comprehensive handbook to an ancient system of movement designed to enhance physical, mental, and spiritual health.

$15.95 US • 224 pages • 7.5 x 9-inch quality paperback • ISBN 978-0-7570-0268-7

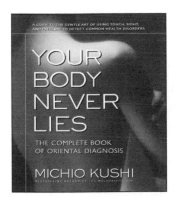

YOUR BODY NEVER LIES
The Complete Book of Oriental Diagnosis
Michio Kushi

Too often, conventional medicine fails to detect illness—especially when it first begins and is easiest to cure. But Oriental diagnosis, an ancient holistic system of knowledge, can often discover physical problems even before they arise. Now *Your Body Never Lies* helps you both understand and use this natural, noninvasive approach to restoring good health.

Your Body Never Lies starts by explaining the principles of Oriental medicine. It then shows you how to detect and understand health problems simply by looking at the mouth, lips, and teeth; eyes; nose, cheeks, and ears; forehead; hair; hands; feet; and skin. Clear diagrams and easy-to-use charts assist you in quickly recognizing signs of illness so that you can begin working toward a state of balanced well-being. Here is a complete guide to Oriental diagnosis, a revolutionary yet centuries-old way to identify and prevent disease while preserving health and harmony.

$16.95 • 184 pages • 7.5 x 9-inch quality paperback • ISBN 978-0-7570-0267-0

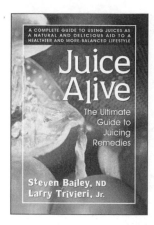

JUICE ALIVE
The Ultimate Guide to Juicing Remedies
Steven Bailey, ND and Larry Trivieri, Jr.

The world of fresh juices offers a powerhouse of antioxidants, vitamins, minerals, and enzymes. The trick is knowing which juices can best serve your needs. In this easy-to-use guide, health experts Dr. Steven Bailey and Larry Trivieri, Jr. tell you everything you need to know to maximize the benefits and tastes of juice.

The book begins with a look at the history of juicing. It then examines the many components that make fresh juice truly good for you—good for weight loss and so much more. Next, it offers practical advice about the types of juices available, as well as buying and storing tips for produce. The second half of the book begins with an important chart that matches up common ailments with the most appropriate juices, followed by over 100 delicious juice recipes. Let *Juice Alive* introduce you to a world bursting with the incomparable tastes and benefits of fresh juice.

$14.95 • 272 pages • 6 x 9-inch quality paperback • ISBN 978-0-7570-0266-3

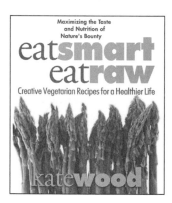

EAT SMART EAT RAW
Creative Vegetarian Recipes for a Healthier Life
Kate Wood

From healing diseases to detoxifying your body, from lowering cholesterol to eliminating excess weight, the many important health benefits derived from a raw vegetarian diet are too important to ignore. However, now there is another compelling reason to go raw—taste! In her new book *Eat Smart, Eat Raw,* cook and health writer Kate Wood not only explains how to get started, but also provides delicious kitchen-tested recipes guaranteed to surprise and delight even the fussiest of eaters.

Eat Smart, Eat Raw begins by explaining the basics of cooking without heat, from choosing the best equipment to stocking your pantry. What follows are twelve recipe chapters filled with truly exceptional dishes, including hearty breakfasts, savory soups, satisfying entrées, and luscious desserts.

$15.95 US • 184 pages • 7.5 x 9-inch quality paperback • ISBN 978-0-7570-0261-8

GOING WILD IN THE KITCHEN
The Fresh & Sassy Tastes of Vegetarian Cooking
Leslie Cerier

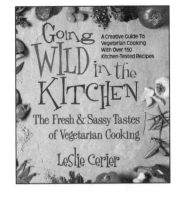

Going Wild in the Kitchen is the first comprehensive global vegetarian cookbook to go beyond the standard organic beans, grains, and vegetables.

In addition to providing helpful cooking tips and techniques, the book contains over 150 kitchen-tested recipes for healthful, taste-tempting dishes—creative masterpieces that contain such unique ingredients as edible flowers; sea vegetables; and wild mushrooms, berries, and herbs. It encourages the creative side of novice and seasoned cooks alike, prompting them to follow their instincts and "go wild" in the kitchen by adding, changing, or substituting ingredients in existing recipes. To help, a wealth of suggestions is found throughout. A list of organic food sources completes this user-friendly cookbook.

$16.95 US • 240 pages • 7.5 x 9-inch quality paperback • ISBN 978-0-7570-0091-1

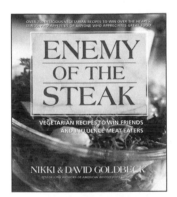

ENEMY OF THE STEAK
Vegetarian Recipes to Win Friends and Influence Meat-Eaters
Nikki and David Goldbeck

Don't blame vegetarians for starting this. Who said "real food for real people"? Aren't asparagus, carrots, and tomatoes every bit as real as . . . that other food? To answer the call to battle, best-selling authors Nikki and David Goldbeck have created a wonderfully tempting new cookbook that offers a wealth of kitchen-tested recipes—recipes that nourish the body, please the palate, and satisfy even the heartiest of appetites.

Enemy of the Steak first presents basic information on vegetarian cooking and stocking the vegetarian pantry. Then eight great chapters offer recipes for breakfast fare; appetizers and hors d'oeuvres; soups; salads; entrées; side dishes; sauces, toppings, and marinades; and desserts. Throughout the book, the Goldbecks have included practical tips and advice on weight loss, disease prevention, and other important topics. They also offer dozens of fascinating facts about why fruits and veggies are so good for you.

A perfect marriage of nutrition and the art of cooking, *Enemy of the Steak* is for everyone who loves a good healthy meal. Simply put, it's great food for smart people. If you have to take sides, you couldn't be in better company.

$16.95 • 248 pages • 7.5 x 9-inch quality paperback • ISBN 978-0-7570-0273-1

GREENS & GRAINS ON THE DEEP BLUE SEA COOKBOOK
Fabulous Vegetarian Cuisine from the Holistic Holiday at Sea Cruises
Sandy Pukel and Mark Hanna

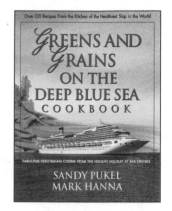

You are invited to come aboard one of America's premier health cruises. Too busy to get away? Even if you can't swim in the ship's pool, you can still enjoy its gourmet cuisine, because natural foods expert Sandy Pukel and master chef Mark Hanna have created *Greens & Grains on the Deep Blue Sea Cookbook*—a titanic collection of the most popular vegetarian dishes served aboard the Holistic Holiday at Sea cruises.

Each of the book's more than 120 recipes is designed to provide not only great taste, but also maximum nutrition. Choose from among an innovative selection of taste-tempting appetizers, soups, salads, entrées, side dishes, and desserts. Easy-to-follow instructions ensure that even novices have superb results. With *Greens & Grains on the Deep Blue Sea Cookbook,* you can enjoy fabulous signature dishes from the Holistic Holiday at Sea cruises in the comfort of your own home.

$16.95 • 160 pages • 7.5 x 9-inch quality paperback • ISBN 978-0-7570-0287-8

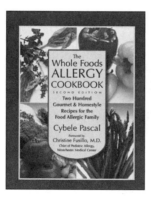

THE WHOLE FOODS ALLERGY COOKBOOK
Two Hundred Gourmet & Homestyle Recipes for the Food Allergic Family
Cybele Pascal

The Whole Foods Allergy Cookbook is the first cookbook to eliminate all eight allergens responsible for ninety percent of food allergies. Each and every dish offered is free of dairy, eggs, wheat, soy, peanuts, tree nuts, fish, and shellfish. You'll find tempting recipes for breakfast pancakes, breads, and cereals; lunch soups, salads, spreads, and sandwiches; dinner entrées and side dishes; dessert puddings, cupcakes, cookies, cakes, and pies; and even after-school snacks ranging from trail mix to pizza and pretzels. Included is a resource guide to organizations that can supply information and support, as well as a shopping guide for hard-to-find items.

If you thought that allergies meant missing out on nutrition, variety, and flavor, think again. With *The Whole Foods Allergy Cookbook,* you'll have both the wonderful taste you want and the radiant health you deserve.

$18.95 • 240 pages • 8 x 10-inch quality paperback • ISBN 978-1-890612-45-0